AGING MY WAY:

Reaching for Bliss

by Daniel Corso

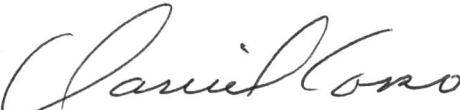

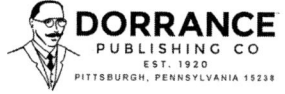

The contents of this work, including, but not limited to, the accuracy of events, people, and places depicted; opinions expressed; permission to use previously published materials included; and any advice given or actions advocated are solely the responsibility of the author, who assumes all liability for said work and indemnifies the publisher against any claims stemming from publication of the work.

The information presented in *Aging My Way: Reaching for Bliss* reveals the author's views, principles, and practices on aging. His way of life, in particular any and all guidelines with regard to maintaining the mind and the body, may not be suitable for everyone, including those with mental and/or physical restrictions and/or disorders. Anyone considering following the guidelines presented herein should first seek the advice of health care professionals.

All Rights Reserved
Copyright © 2018 by Daniel Corso

No part of this book may be reproduced or transmitted, downloaded, distributed, reverse engineered, or stored in or introduced into any information storage and retrieval system, in any form or by any means, including photocopying and recording, whether electronic or mechanical, now known or hereinafter invented without permission in writing from the publisher.

Dorrance Publishing Co
585 Alpha Drive
Pittsburgh, PA 15238
Visit our website at *www.dorrancebookstore.com*

ISBN: 978-1-4809-4949-2
eISBN: 978-1-4809-4926-3

Acknowledgements

My lady soul Betty: for your undying support and loyalty when I needed it most;

Mom and dad: for your loving guidance and selfless standard;

Cousin David Balducci: for your courageous model and constant reassurance;

Class of '64 "Brother Rats" of Big Mike: for your support during hard times;

An unknown Roman Catholic priest: for your homily, a defining moment in my life.

Those flashes of pleasure, sometimes bliss,
Assuage moments of pain, occasional sorrow,
Grateful for reassurance from our past,
We remain faithful about tomorrow.

Introduction

The process of moving through the various stages of life engenders involuntary physical and mental transformations that trigger the need to make lifestyle adjustments. None is more powerful than the changes imposed by the senior phase. It can take away our purpose in life, leaving a void that needs to be filled. To complicate matters, thanks to advances in healthcare and information technology, many of us are living longer, healthier lives. To those of us so blessed, it is important not to squander such a valuable, irreplaceable opportunity.

When I entered the senior stage of life, I was in good physical, mental and financial condition. Still, I was unprepared to make the adjustment. I didn't have a plan on how to use my time. This created a degree of stress in my life, which had the potential to be devastating.

Thanks to an unexpected boost, which proved to be a defining moment in my life, I eventually developed a set of balanced, all-inclusive practices that greatly improved my quality of life. I am now content and thriving in my mid-seventies, and I look forward to what life has in store for me as I reach for bliss in Eternal Life.

Aging My Way: Reaching for Bliss was written to share these ideologies with other seniors and those approaching the final phase of life, hoping to enrich those that read it.

With kind regards, I am,
Daniel Corso

Table of Contents

1. A new era dawns 1
2. Precedents 8
3. Concern-based behavior 17
4. Principles 23
5. Wealth 25
6. Work 32
7. Morality 41
8. Spirituality 48
9. Fitness 58
10. Legacy 66
11. Transitioning 74
12. Practice: Prepare for Eternal Life 89
13. Practice: Engage life head on 99
14. Practice: Reconcile the past 114
15. Practice: Stay fit 129
16. Marching forward 138

Chapter 1
A new era dawns

According to a national media release, researchers reported the number of Americans ages 65 and older increased tenfold in the last century, and the elderly are living longer, in more comfort and in better health than ever before. This should not surprise any senior that has compared their station in life to that of their parents and grandparents at the same age. Still, it's comforting to know that folks being paid for compiling actuarial data have confirmed our observations. Certainly, the statistics delight everyone, not just seniors. We expend a significant portion of our resources to prolong and enrich our lives, and this pursuit is being attained. That said, like with many things in life, there is a secondary effect. The evolution of our lifespan begs a question: what should we do with the extra time?

Going through the various stages leading up to that glorious stage called retirement, our plates were jam-packed with meaningful items that demanded our attention. The list seemed endless. As soon as we scratched an item off the list, one or more would replace it. We would wake up many mornings with full agendas of important matters. Although we were living in a free society, our lives were regulated to a great extent by our list. However, the situation would radically change in retirement. The list shortened significantly and abruptly, setting us free from many of the responsibilities constraining us. Retirement created a void in our lives, one that needed to be filled. This evolution presented a wonderful opportunity, and it left us with a choice. Should we take full advantage of our gift or squander it?

Unquestionably, with freedom comes responsibility. Life is not solely about existing, but about attaining happiness in the process. The Founding Fathers clearly understood this, and they made certain the concept was expressed in this phrase from our Declaration of Independence: "Life, liberty and the *pursuit of happiness*." Although modern-day Americans have been gifted liberty and protracted longevity, two of the elements referenced by Thomas Jefferson, we do not necessarily have the third. Mr. Jefferson associated *pursuit* with *happiness* for a reason. It is an emotion that comes and goes, one that is impossible to corral. We are constantly chasing it. Furthermore, as we move into and through the senior phase of life, our drive begins to wane and so does our energy to pursue anything.

When I reached the senior phase of life, my general health and probability of having a long life were better than average. Nevertheless, I was less than passionate about my life, and even less about my future. The gaps between those treasured moments of contentment were widening. I was missing something. After taking stock of myself, I decided to adjust some of my principles that were impacting my state of mind. I needed to be more balanced. It didn't occur immediately, but I eventually adopted a lifestyle that provided contentment on a more dependable basis. And as a result, my life improved drastically. I am now thriving in my mid-seventies.

THE LONGEVITY TREND

As previously noted, Americans are living longer and better than their ancestors. And this is probably the state of affairs in other civilized countries around the world. The evolution is a byproduct of scientific advancements in health care coupled with a surge in communication and information technology. Accordingly, a noticeable shift in the architype for seniors is in progress. The age threshold has become a moving target, one that seems to be inching higher and higher. Additionally, this trend is unlikely to discontinue or slow in the foreseeable future. Instead, it is more likely that new scientific breakthroughs are on the horizon, which will cause our health and longevity to improve even more.

The effect is being felt

Scientists have warned the world about the magnitude of a global warming trend in our climate. The human race doesn't know whether or not this alarm is meritorious because we have yet to observe a noticeable detrimental consequence. However, this isn't the case with rising longevity. Americans are feeling a forceful economic ramification. Prolonged existence is one of the contributors to the national debt and the threatened state of Medicare and Social Security, those hard-earned monies contributed by millions of Americans over long periods of time. This raises a controversial question: if seniors could make adjustments to their lifestyles that would moderate the problem, should they? In a free society like America's, this is a matter of individual choice, as it should be. Nonetheless, protracted longevity is an issue that can no longer be ignored.

Valuable or valueless?

As I went through life, I made certain to observe people older than me. I wanted to learn from them and get a glimpse of my future. It was apparent that the process of aging entailed change. One of the changes is the state of retirement, a topic this book explores in some detail later.

Leaving the workforce was an expected byproduct of surviving to age 65; society generally viewed seniors as unable to make significant contributions any longer. Seniors were considered to have lost much of their value. However, I have been noticing a subtle shift in the underlying reason for the stereotype. Not only were seniors living longer, but also many were in decent physical and mental condition. Thus, the premise upon which this culture was founded is weakening. Can healthy seniors contribute more to society? Yes, but to do so demands altering the perception of who they were into the reality of who they are.

Is a cultural shift in progress?
Most of my acquaintances, Baby Boomers that I have known for decades, hoped to live long enough to retire. If and when they attained their goal, they wanted to possess sufficient financial assets to enjoy the final phase of their lives. Many of them had set their retirement age target at 65 or earlier, a reasonable track given the mortality data when they began their careers. However, because the life expectancy of people rose during that period, the financial strategy wasn't always appropriate. Not all of them stopped working at 65, and in some cases the decision was financially driven.

In other situations, working past 65 was not an economic necessity. Several of them, who are in their mid-seventies and who have been successful entrepreneurs most of their adult lives, have disregarded their economic ability not to work. They continue to be industrious members of society, and so have some very prominent people in America. For example, while I was working to get this book published, the 2016 United States presidential election was underway. The two main candidates vying to take up residency in the White House were wealthy seniors; they could have spurned seeking the office to pursue lives of luxury, but they chose not to do so. If we could dig deep into their souls and bare the truth, we would find a powerful driving force. Perhaps it was a hunger for power or a desire to attain a place in history or the need to improve their country or some combination thereof. Irrespective of their reasons, the candidates were willing to make a huge personal sacrifice. Are these examples a microcosm of a shift in the culture of seniors? The sample size is so small that it is almost invisible. Nevertheless, if a cultural shift is in progress, it would be beneficial to society.

Financial plans are necessary, but risky

Many people look forward to the day when they will be free from work and similar responsibilities, which will allow them to devote all or most of their energy to addressing bucket lists, enjoying exotic destinations, managing financial portfolios, dining in exclusive restaurants and like activities. To engage in such lifestyles requires sufficient money, of course, which is the primary reason so much attention is focused on seniors being financially successful and stable. This book addresses a number of important issues related to happiness, but it does not offer advice on financial investment and/or management. There are countless authorities earning handsome livings hawking those services.

As an aside, like most of my peers, I engage a professional for that task. Still, I have misgivings. Having a financial plan is much better than nothing, but there are a number of uncontrollable risks associated with them. It is difficult to make reliable economic forecasts, especially when the future exceeds more than a few years as it does with most financial plans. Nobody can possibly predict and/or quantify all of the variables critical to these strategies. Although historical information has often proven to be a reliable predictor of the future, the modern era is a different age, one abounding with danger. The world has never before accumulated the magnitude of debt it is burdened with today, which could affect the cost of living, the value of currencies, global economic stability, political power, wars and the like. Could indebtedness eventually make the American government insolvent? An answer to this frightening, provocative question is well outside the boundaries of this book. However, it would be unwise to dismiss the possibility as ludicrous. If history has proven anything, it is that governments eventually struggle to remain stable, and the underlying reason has always been economic. The government of the United States – *We the People* for those of us that remember and respect the Constitution – is on shaky financial ground these days. At the time this book was written, America's indebtedness was approaching 20 trillion dollars and growing. That's *20 trillion dollars* or *20 x 1 million x 1 million dollars*! If and when the debt is called, what would happen? And I believe the perception that our government is economically unstable is one of the underlying reasons for robust gun sales in this great country of ours.

A HOLISTIC, BALANCED APPROACH TO AGING

Instead of financial planning, this book concentrates on other important aspects of life that can greatly impact an individual's state of well-being. These will be presented in the form of principles and practices that have proven invaluable in improving my overall quality of life. Regrettably, I entered the senior phase of life with a narrow, purely monetary and self-centered outlook, which produced stress instead of contentment. Although it took time, I eventually developed and applied a holistic, balanced approach to life.

One of the principles that will be presented is spirituality, a key factor in an individual's overall well-being. When I reached the senior phase of life, my spiritual tank was nearly on empty. I believed in God, but I was snubbing my Christian upbringing and my Roman Catholic faith. Because I was mostly operating on fumes, I had to make an adjustment to my spiritual approach. And when I did, the quality of my life improved.

Fitness is another principle that will be advanced. I once overheard a senior remark, "Growing old isn't for sissies." I can't dispute the truth behind the witticism, nor will I attempt to do so. After all, the mind and the body are fragile; they aren't designed to last forever, and there is no Fountain of Youth, as Ponce de Leon discovered when he failed to find vitality-restoring waters. As the years pass, the erosion of time causes everything to weaken, and this is especially true of that intricate composite of biological matter known as the human body. It will eventually reach a point when it breaks down. And when it fails, quality of life tends to degrade very, very quickly. That said, many seniors haven't reached that point and may actually be healthy enough to maintain an appropriate overall condition, both physically and mentally. Individuals that take the necessary measures to do so tend to improve their quality of life. And this certainly applies to all adults, not just seniors. Because I was fortunate to be in better-than-average health, I adjusted my routine to help me reach and sustain a good level of fitness for my age and condition. This proactive choice has produced excellent results for me.

In addition to spirituality and fitness, this book explores and endorses principles on wealth, work, morality and legacy, all of which shape the realistic practices that I use to attain happiness on a more consistent basis. Prior to presenting them, it is important to first lay a solid foundation.

CHAPTER 2
Precedents

There are a number of precedents that relate directly to the principles and practices that will be developed later in this book. Let's get right to them.

HEALTH

Many, if not all humans eventually come to understand that good health is the most treasured asset in life, far more valuable than wealth. Why is this true? There are two compelling reasons.

First, it is effectively impossible to enjoy the benefits of wealth without good health. When we are in pain from and/or we are afflicted with one or more debilitating physical or mental condition, we cannot use wealth, no matter great, to fully experience the joys of life. Consequently, in order to maximize the life experience, good health is more essential than wealth.

Second, good health is impossible to purchase at any price. Irrespective of how much wealth a person has amassed, they either have good health or they don't. Wealth, on the other hand, is only a commodity, albeit an important one. Humans are attracted to wealth because it: brings a sense of security in the game of survival, assuages some of life's pain and enables gratifying pursuits. Otherwise, in and of itself, wealth is meaningless. If one doesn't have it today, they have an opportunity to attain it tomorrow. Conversely, if one has it today, they are at risk to lose it tomorrow.

One of my relatives, who is now deceased, once said to me, "I'd give everything I have to feel like I did when I was 25." He was a wealthy senior at the time. Although he wasn't handicapped or suffering, he didn't feel good and he was losing his zeal for life. It wasn't what he said that struck me, but the conviction with which he expressed it. He blurted it out quite unexpectedly in a casual social setting. More importantly, his facial expression told me that he was deadly serious. Given the opportunity to make a swap, he would have gladly traded his hefty holdings to recapture the energy and the physical and mental condition he possessed in his youth. He had spent most of his life working hard and investing, but his fortune was unable to provide what he held dearest. Thus, the wealth he had accumulated lost its value. Is my relative's perspective uncommon? I think not, especially as we approach the end of our lives.

Although wealth will be addressed at length in Chapter 5, this is a good place to interject a comment that my mom once made on the subject: "Money is only good if it's used when it's needed." Dismissing the importance of money sitting in a bank, she only valued money when it was exchanged for something essential, something that improved quality of life. And if money wasn't used when needed, it was worthless. Being young at the time that I heard her remark, her sage viewpoint didn't impress me as much as it does now.

PRECEDENT 1:
Good health is more valuable than wealth.

LONGEVITY
Similar to good health, longevity can't be purchased at any price.

Let's put the concept of time into perspective. Scientific evidence shows that Earth, the third planet from the sun, has been in existence for billions of years. That's right, *b* as in *billion*. And this wondrous marvel we call Earth contains millions of species, of which the human race is but one. Assessing the average human life span in that context, we don't need scientists or statistical models to establish the fact that an individual's longevity is miniscule in the grand scheme of nature.

Does this indicate that our lives are insignificant? Of course it doesn't. However, it does show that humans have very little of that coveted, precious possession called time to accomplish anything significant. And for Christians that believe in Eternal Life, it implies that God gave humans a very small window of opportunity to save their souls. Consequently, what human beings and particularly Christians do with their time on Earth becomes critically important.

PRECEDENT 2:
Longevity is more valuable than wealth, and it should not be squandered.

QUALITY OF LIFE
Given the choice, would a reasonable human opt to live one year in perfect contentment or ten years in hopeless misery? This is, obviously, a hypothetical question posed to establish a point: going through the motions of breathing for the sake of breathing is far less important than breathing to enjoy one's time.

I recall spending a pleasant evening with my cousin Chris. After consuming a delightful meal, we made a couple of highballs and moved to his patio. I took a sip from my glass, which contained a couple of ounces of Macallan 12-year-old single malt Scotch Whiskey over ice. Then I looked at him and quoted a line I had once heard, "All we can do is tie this."

He replied, "I couldn't have said it any better."

At that precise moment in time, we were perfectly content. Certainly, the world offered finer foods and beverages, but our meal and libations were utterly satisfying to us. More importantly, so was the company, the conversation and the pleasant breeze that was stirring. We could not have improved on the moment we were experiencing. Perfection is perfection. Contentment is contentment. There is no progressive scale. When one reaches that highly-valued state of mind, maintaining it becomes the challenge.

We spend a significant amount of time pursuing objectives that often define our lives and the perception others have of us. As we move forward, we long to achieve contentment. In one way or another, we pursue this subjective, elusive emotion. And what satisfies one individual may leave another person wanting. There is no perfect formula, a one-size-fits-all plan. Nevertheless, everyone needs to be on a pathway to contentment, without which quality of life will deteriorate.

PRECEDENT 3:
Contentment is more valuable than longevity.

RELATIONSHIPS
While it's possible for humans acting on their own to acquire food and shelter, they will obtain it more readily, and in all probability better, with the help of others. Thus, because we need each other to prosper, establishing and maintaining wholesome relationships with others is an important factor in attaining contentment.

When I attended and graduated from Virginia Tech, it had an ROTC program and a strong "Rat System" for incoming freshmen. During those intense days and months adjusting to the burdens of academics and the "Rat System," my "Brother Rats" and I formed tight bonds. Few of us, if any, would have been able to stay the course alone. We were forced to learn and practice the valuable skill called teamwork. Through the years and the decades that ensued, long after we tossed our caps into the air at our graduation ceremony, many of us kept in touch. We never forgot the times we depended on each other so profoundly. And I would venture to state this is still the case today at any military college with a strong "Rat System."

Not only can establishing and maintaining healthy relationships increase the odds of surviving, it can improve one's inner peace. But not everyone is inclined to be peaceful. Individuals characterized by a warrior mentality are inclined to be judgmental and confrontational, often dramatically.

Human relationships are extremely fragile, almost too delicate at times. Once they have been fractured, mending them can be very, very difficult. And it's practically impossible to go through life without being annoyed by others from time to time. Close relationships are particularly vulnerable because of frequency of contact and demanding, sometimes unrealistic expectations. Marriages are perhaps the best example. It is a fact that marriage vows, like all partnership agreements, will be pressured at some point. Commitment seems to be a lost principle in modern society; self-centered behavior seems to be much more prevalent. When divorce occurs, breakups can be intensely confrontational and sometimes violent.

It is often astounding what a new and better outlook can bring to a relationship. A family situation with which I am familiar comes to mind. The father of one of my relatives had a well-deserved reputation for being extremely self-centered. The father consistently placed his needs and wants above everyone, even his wife and children. After the children became adults, one of his sons harbored resentment for a very long time. As the decades passed, the son purged the bitterness and found forgiveness. Wanting a better relationship, the son accepted the father's good and bad traits. They reconciled and found peace with each other. Later, the father came to live with his son, and he was treated respectfully until he died.

PRECEDENT 4:

Establishing and maintaining wholesome relationships empowers contentment.

CHANGE

Benjamin Franklin originated the cliché, "In this world nothing can be said to be certain, expect death and taxes." Every time I see or hear this quote being used, the person is usually emphasizing the barb on taxes. For me, the more salient but less-heralded point of his remark is that *change is an inevitable part of life*. When Mr. Franklin wisely coined the phrase, he succinctly struck the nail directly on the head. Life, my friends, is all about change. Those that can adjust well usually do well. Those that can't are likely disposed to have problems.

There are emotional ups and downs attached to changes in our lives. They can be extremely unsettling if and when they impact our sense of security – tornado watch in the area, terrorism at an elementary school, investment loss, job loss, death of loved ones and similar troubling events. On the other hand, positive changes such as business success, achieving recognition or establishing new, wholesome relationships tend to be very uplifting.

Whichever way change impacts us, an absolute truth is that nothing remains the same forever. Change, positive or negative, with or without anyone's permission, is inevitable. In some respects, it makes life much more interesting.

PRECEDENT 5:
Change is unescapable.

CONTROL
Humans attempt to control everything in their environment that directly influences their lives. Trying to micromanage life is quite natural, but it can be extremely challenging and frustrating; this is particularly true when attempting to control the actions of people.

For instance, society utilizes traffic signals, lane markings, speed limits, signage and the like in the hopes of making travel safer. However, such devices are anything but a guarantee of safety. The willingness of people to comply with society's laws is a huge factor, and some are prone to be disobedient. Others are simply negligent. When using public thoroughfares, it is imperative to pay strict attention to what others are doing, not what they should be doing.

While it may be true that humans exercise a degree of control over some aspects of their lives, we exert no command over many of the important things that affect us. From moment to moment, it is difficult to predict what may happen in life. For example, we have no control over death, evil, some diseases and climatic disasters, all of which can arise with little or no warning and can significantly alter the lives of people in a harsh way. Hence, we are really out of control much of the time, irrespective of what we believe.

PRECEDENT 6:
Humans exercise no control over many significant events.

PURPOSE & PASSION
That strong, almost uncontrollable desire known as passion is the human trait of the spirit that enables us to embrace life enthusiastically.

And based on my observations, those with passion extract much more from life than those lacking it. Thus, it is one of the keys to happiness.

However, in order to acquire passion, humans need purpose. By definition, purpose is the reason that something is done or exists, the inner characteristic of humans that keeps us moving forward. Expressing this in a different way, purpose is the resource that instills passion.

The motivator that compels humans to want to live is an inborn survival instinct. However, living just to survive is an unacceptable approach to being a member of the human race. Life should not be about breathing and taking up space. It should be about enjoying the gift to the fullest, while returning something of value in exchange. When we rise to start a new day, we should be enthusiastic about accomplishing something that gives us pride and joy. At the end of each day, the opportunity to achieve anything meaningful that day is gone forever.

Regrettably, attaining a *meaningful* purpose can be problematic for seniors, even for those that find themselves fortunate enough to be healthy. The process of aging slowly takes away the substantive things that once motivated us to be passionate: raising offspring, socializing with family and friends, developing careers, being a provider, achieving wealth and so forth. These important roles in life are eventually displaced by insignificant functions and attending funerals, which can be a breeding ground for loneliness and depression. It is not unusual for those approaching the senior phase of life or in it to lose interest in achieving meaningful goals. We tend to look backward at what we did, not look forward at what we are about to do. And at some point, seniors come to understand that the materialistic goals they once aspired to attain are really transient in nature and relatively unimportant. Nevertheless, becoming a senior is not in and of itself mutually exclusive to having purpose and passion. It is matter of choice.

The following quote in italics was authored by Joseph Epstein, essayist, short-story writer and editor: *"We do not choose to be born. We do not choose our parents. We do not choose our historical epoch, or the country of our birth, or the immediate circumstances of our upbringing. We do not, most of us, choose to die nor do we choose the time or conditions of our death. But within all this realm of choicelessness, we do choose how we shall live: courageously or in cowardice, honorably or dishonorably, with purpose or adrift. We decide what is important and what is trivial in life. We decide that what makes us significant is either what we do or what we refuse to do. But no matter how indifferent the universe may be to our choices and decisions, these choices and decisions are ours to make. We decide. We choose. And as we decide and choose, so are our lives formed. In the end, forming our own destiny is what ambition is about."*

This declaration perfectly, concisely summarizes the all-important outcome attached to choice. It applies to everyone, of course, including seniors. As we progress through life, the meaningful goals that we embrace are a derivative of a conscientious, deliberate decision process. As Mr. Epstein so powerfully states: "We decide. We choose. And as we decide and choose, so are our lives formed." And should we make the conscientious choice to live without any significant purpose, we are set adrift. This is not the best way to go through life…at any age. We should always aspire to hold meaningful goals, which have the power to keep the fire of passion burning inside us.

PRECEDENT 7:
Humans need a meaningful purpose.

CHAPTER 3
Concern-based behavior

It is always interesting to observe the stimuli for human behavior, and certainly concern can be a key force in an individual's actions. When writing this book, I briefly examined my concern-based motivators as I went through life; I discovered they had changed significantly, and one of them eventually became dominant during the last phase of my life. This chapter is devoted to that self-study.

Using a baseball analogy, which should be familiar to almost everyone, I divided life into four distinct phases – (1) Childhood Phase (home plate to 1st base); (2) Adolescent Phase (1st base to 2nd base); (3) Adult Phase (2nd base to 3rd base); and (4) Senior Phase (3rd base to home plate). This works extremely well because baseball imitates life in many ways. In order to score, ballplayers must first take a position in the batters' box at home plate; there they have a clean slate, like a newborn with an unblemished record. An infant will use any available resource to survive and grow in order to advance through the other stages of life. Similarly, ballplayers use their skills, hoping to reach their goal: progressing around each base and returning to home plate. And like humans making the trek through life, ballplayers can be put out anytime, anywhere as they attempt to make the circuit.

As an aside, I became interested in baseball as a child, largely due to the influence of my dad, an avid fan of the New York Yankees. Like my dad, I became a Yankee supporter as a result of a unique gift he gave me. Thanks to an inside connection, he learned which hotel the Yankees would use during a stay in Washington DC for a series with the Senators, and he made certain I was in position to meet the players. One or two at a time, as the Yankees – Yogi Berra, Bill Skowron, Whitey Ford, et al. – entered the lobby on the way to the hotel restaurant for breakfast, I asked them to autograph my baseball. All of them willingly obliged. When I noticed that Mickey Mantle and Billy Martin had escaped my blockade, I hunted them down in the restaurant; while they were signing my ball, they bought me a coke and asked me to sit with them. I gave that baseball, the most treasured article from my past, to one of my grandsons. And he also received the story of the experience with my dad and the big-heartedness of those legendary ballplayers, many of whom earned a place in the National Baseball Hall of Fame in Cooperstown, New York.

With that digression out of the way, the following is a recap of the concern-based drivers that influenced my behavior as I toured the bases of life.

(1) Childhood Phase (home plate to 1st base) – In this early stage of life, I recall only one concern that impacted my behavior. It was a fixation on the danger that venomous snakes and insects posed, which was a byproduct of my lifestyle. The expensive gifts and toys that are heaped upon children today were non-existent for me and most of the kids I knew; thus, my best friend and I invented our entertainment. We spent quite a bit of time roaming through a forest bordering the Chickahominy Swamp, where we learned about nature and potentially harmful wildlife such as copperhead snakes and Black Widow spiders. After

learning about the damage these marvels of nature could inflict on human beings, they immediately gained my respect. To insure my bed had not been invaded by one of these creatures, I remember thoroughly examining it before retiring. Given that my home was safe, this was completely unnecessary. Nevertheless, this concern-based ritual stayed with me through most of my childhood before eventually fading away.

(2) Adolescent Phase (1st base to 2nd base) – In this stage of my life, when I became aware of myself and developed self-esteem, I adopted new concern-based dispositions. The most dominant one was my fear of failure. I'm not certain about its origin, but my actions were controlled by it. During my high school years, it drove me to strive for academic excellence and to perform summer jobs well. And I was also preoccupied with being accepted by my peers; I wanted them to like and respect me. At the tender age of seventeen, I graduated from high school and trudged off to college. Although this was a tough adjustment at first, my obsession not to fail drove me to work exceptionally hard in the pursuit of a mechanical engineering degree and a commission as a 2nd Lieutenant in the United States Army, both of which I accomplished in four years.

(3) Adult Phase (2nd base to 3rd base) – As a young adult, my sense of self-importance and self-assurance began to surge. I was confident in my ability to handle almost any situation, including circumstances that I encountered during my brief military career as a combat engineer. After being assigned to Vietnam, I was trained in the importance of personal security. I remained vigilant with at least one locked and loaded weapon at all times, hoping this would protect me. This was necessary, of course, but it did not afford protection from hostile sniper fire, incoming mortar shells, booby-traps and a variety of other potential

dangers. The differentiator between being uninjured or being killed or maimed was fate. Some of my college classmates were less fortunate than me. In 1965, one of my "Brother Rats," 1st Lieutenant Bill Webb, was ambushed and killed at Long Binh, which was in the same region as my location, a village called Cu Chi. Another, Major Bobby Edmunds, was shot down and killed in 1968 over North Vietnam. As my tour of 'Nam drew to a close, I became extremely careful. At the crack of dawn one morning, a few days before I was scheduled to hop on a helicopter to start my journey to the United States, I was part of a patrol to check our encampment defenses. As I was moving through the danger zone, a thought crossed my mind: during the night, when our ability to spot the Viet Cong was severely hampered, the enemy could have infiltrated the perimeter wire and planted land mines. Driven by this spontaneous notion, I immediately began to tread even more guardedly.

When I was back in the United States, I met my partner in life. After we married, I fathered two children. As responsible men do, I assumed the role of providing for my family and took the duty very seriously. After working for several employers, I cofounded an engineering business with two partners. Although my sense of self-importance and self-confidence were diminishing a bit, they were still dominant factors in my behavior. During this stage of my life, I was prideful, especially about my family and my business. Driven to see them excel and fearful that they wouldn't, I was willing to work extremely hard.

At that point in my life, I also had a health-based concern. I had witnessed the ravages of lung cancer on a dear family member, and I was determined not to fall prey to this disease. As a result of that fear, coupled with my wife's asthmatic condition, I gave up smoking cigarettes, a habit that I acquired in the military.

(4) Senior Phase (3rd base to home plate) – The concern-based obsessions that dominated my behavior during the first three phases of my life were either gone or they had greatly diminished. However, new concerns developed and replaced the old ones.

I became troubled about the way of life for the generations that I will leave behind. Unfortunately, I had to accept the fact that I was essentially powerless to affect the future or to make national and global problems disappear. Still, it's impossible to overlook them. The world is an awful mess, thanks to leaders that have repeatedly displayed a propensity for corruption and/or immorality and/or ineptness and/or barbarism. I have frequently admonished myself, "Did I do all that I could to prevent the current state of affairs?" I would like to be able answer that question with a resounding, "Yes," but in all honesty, I will carry some guilt to my grave.

The modern world is much more dangerous than the one I remember growing up. We cannot assume that we'll be safe, even inside America's borders. It's no longer fashionable for thugs and political criminals to enact evil like they did in the past. Random violence in the form of vicious home invasions, acts of terrorism and kidnappings with malicious intent are the latest tactics of evil-doers, who prefer to ambush unsuspecting, peaceful people without warning; malevolence of this nature can surface anywhere, anytime. Although this type of threat wasn't within my sphere of influence, it did impact my behavior. I employ security technology and I maintain weapons on hand. I know how to use them and I am committed to do so, if and when necessary. I also caution family members to be wary of the dangers lurking in the world, and I have provided arms to some of my older grandchildren.

My most dominant concern is that I haven't met God's expectations when I came out of my mother's womb, the moment when I first stepped into the batters' box. Every human I have ever known, including me, dislikes uncertainty. I want to score a run, but I'm unclear if I've done enough to earn it. I will no longer take risks that the Bible is wrong or simply a hoax. If there really is a Promised Land where bliss exists and lasts forever – and you will learn later that I believe there is and why I believe it – I want to be included. Therefore, I had to significantly alter my routine in the hopes of reaching bliss in Eternal Life.

Summary

While I was rounding the bases, my concern-based behavior was undergoing a transformation and I believe for the better. In order to be capable of distinguishing between what was truly important and what was meaningless, I had to undergo a maturation process. In the final phase of life, the concerns of my youth had been supplanted by deep, meaningful issues like the future of the world that I'll leave behind and my status with God. It was too late for me to make the world a better place, but it wasn't too late to try to save my soul. Looking at myself from outside the box, I came to grips with who I had been and who I wanted to be. It was a self-initiated examination of conscience, which made me realize that I needed to change my behavior. I would have to improve my routine by shedding my ego and becoming more selfless; otherwise, I could never be comfortable that I had done my very best to satisfy God.

Chapter 4
Principles

Principles, sometimes referred to as values or ideologies, are human views that underpin behavior; this topic is introduced here for a very good reason. Values not only influence behavior, but they also can be a source of contentment. As we age, it becomes increasingly important to adopt and maintain righteous principles. Not only do we depend on them for strength, our Creator insists that we live by them, making them a portal to Eternal Life.

Regrettably, not all humans are inclined to champion righteousness as a way of life. A percentage of the populace actually subscribes to evil ideologies. Those falling into this category lack a conscience and have no misgivings about malevolent behavior. In fact, they prefer it. In the past we have seen this clearly demonstrated in the form of Adolf Hitler, Idi Amin, Osama bin Laden, John Wayne Gacy and countless others like them. Relying on the regularity with which history has documented the existence of savages like these, it would appear the world will always breed clones.

Fortunately, these kinds of soulless creatures are exceptions. The vast majority of humans are steered by that wonderful gift from God called the human conscience, which allows us to differentiate between moral and immoral behavior. It follows that principled-centered behavior based on the human conscience is generally accepted by society and, more importantly, by our Creator.

However, the human conscience has a gray zone between the extremes of moral and immoral behavior, which will be covered extensively in Chapter 7. Individuals, who are generally regarded to be moral, can exhibit fundamentally dissimilar behavior in identical situations. Some will always behave with absolute integrity, irrespective of the personal outcome. Others will justify minor infringements or simply ignore their conscience when tempted to better themselves, especially if nobody will know. For example, I'll use this golf analogy. To a great extent, golf is a game of self-regulation, which also mirrors life. Most amateur golfers are familiar with the key rules of the game, but not everyone abides by all of them, all of the time. Some players are inclined to improve their lie (condition of the golf ball at rest) and/or miscount strokes, which are contrary to the rules. In effect, they're cheating . . . not only their competitors but themselves. Years ago, I participated in a foursome match, in which money was being wagered. As one of the players placed his ball on the first tee to start the match, another player asked the group, "Are we playing *real* golf today?" He knew there was a chance one or two would break the rules, and he did not wish to be improperly disadvantaged.

In addition to the examination of morality in Chapter 7, principles on wealth, work, spirituality, fitness and legacy, which have been significant in shaping my state of mind during the final stage of my life, will be expounded upon in subsequent chapters.

Chapter 5
Wealth

We are driven to seek wealth because material goods are essential for our survival. Having control over a stockpile of resources in a world full of unknowns is reassuring, particularly to offset the unpredictability of the future. The more goods an individual has, the longer they should be able to endure. And the opposite is also true. The less an individual has, the more vulnerable they are. Thus, there is a direct correlation between an individual's prosperity and their sense of security, making wealth one of the factors in contentment. But does wealth, in and of itself, produce happiness?

Prior to addressing this question, let me set the record straight on my view of wealth. It's human nature to be attracted to money and the things it can obtain, and I'm human. As with most people, the idea of having plenty of money in my pocket, a surplus of cash in the bank, real estate, stocks, bonds and precious metals appeals to me. I also like the smell and look of a new car, the feel of new clothes and so forth. To say otherwise would be a lie. However, being enticed by wealth and loving it are vastly different. I *like* it. I don't *love* it. Consequently, the epicenter of my life isn't wealth. And I don't choose my friends based on their net worth. I choose them based on their integrity and how they treat others. I'm also not envious of individuals that have more than me. I'm happy for them. And I'm also open to helping individuals less fortunate than me, which I have proven on many occasions.

My view on wealth allows me to look at it objectively, and I will. Many humans mistakenly focus too much attention on wealth, believing it is the most important accomplishment in life, the thing that brings happiness. If only life was that simple. It isn't. In fact, there are a number of problems that can be associated with wealth.

One of them is stress. The basic nature of riches, a great quantity of which is the definition of wealth, is transitory. Wealth isn't permanent. It is subject to change, and it sometimes disappears. Once an individual acquires it, they are challenged with the responsibility of safeguarding it and hopefully growing it. Hence, wealth can engender a certain degree of anxiety. It must be protected from those ready, willing and capable of seizing it. This threat has always been a problem, but it is becoming more widespread in modern society with technological advances in the form of computers, communications, the Internet and social media. Intellectual thieves from all over the world are concocting ways to prey upon unprepared targets. Seniors, most of whom are living on fixed incomes, cannot afford to become victims of such crimes. And old forms of white-collared thievery continue to be serious dangers today. Pedigreed swindlers, who are motivated solely to enrich themselves, can be masked under the pretext of legitimate businesses and stations in life. We have seen many examples of individuals in positions of trust who have granted themselves outrageous salaries and/or perks and/or simply embezzled funds. This type of larceny has been uncovered in a variety of charitable organizations, legal entities and financial companies. While I was writing this book, a major bank was forced to fire thousands of employees for defrauding customers. It takes significant restraint for trusting investors not to retaliate strongly against cold-hearted, calculating scam artists that steal from them.

There is no doubt about greed, an intense selfish desire for wealth, being a source of evil, which is the point of 1 Timothy 6:10 in the New Testament: "For the love of money is the root of all evil: which while some coveted after, they have erred from the faith, and pierced themselves through with many sorrows." Most of us can probably recite stories about money and/or the things money can purchase being the cause of broken relationships. It can, of course, also lead to abusive and violent behavior. If wealth is the key to happiness, why have a number of lottery winners become the victim of a drug overdose, suicide, home invasion, lawsuit or murder?

There can also be another negative outcome. When humans that place wealth on a pedestal set materialistic goals and fail, they usually experience great disappointment, and sometimes even depression. In effect, they become victims of self-inflicted wounds. And should they set materialistic goals and succeed, the euphoria is almost always short-lived. Financial markets are a good example. As they undergo up and down cycles, it's difficult for investors not to experience emotional highs and lows as the markets swing.

During my life, I have known a few people that were truly in love with money and the things it can bring. After some had achieved substantial wealth, when they became older and wiser and understood their mortality, they became increasingly disinterested in their riches. Their material portfolio failed to deliver a state of happiness, much less bliss. Observing these situations led me to conclude that acquiring and hoarding possessions is not the pathway to happiness.

Reinforcing this supposition is a lengthy list of wealthy luminaries that, with little or no warning, killed themselves. Some were drug-related deaths, unintentional or not. Others were definitely planned. We don't need Sherlock Holmes to get to the bottom of the problem. The trigger for these mind-boggling events was unhappiness. Unable to achieve and/or to perpetuate contentment, they were anything but the personalities they projected in public. Somewhere deep inside themselves, despite the images they portrayed, they needed more from life than they were receiving. In the end, their worldly possessions – mansions, garages packed with luxury cars, jewelry boxes stuffed with precious gems, public acclaim and the like – left them frustrated and wanting. To attain and maintain peace of mind, there needs to be more, something more powerful than finite possessions. For those able to draw their last breath in absolute accord with the world and themselves, their belongings will have little or nothing to do with them achieving it.

And then there is the unusual case of Roseto, a borough located in Northampton County, Pennsylvania. The Italian inhabitants had an exceptionally low heart disease rate. This defied what should have happened given their eating and drinking habits. The men even smoked Italian stogie cigars. The community also had no crime and few applications for social assistance. This borough became the subject of a study, which concluded that the good health in the close-knit community was related to the stress-free, cohesive lifestyle, a phenomenon called the Roseto effect. However, the situation would eventually change. As the populace assimilated into the affluent culture of mainstream America, the people became less healthy. Saying it differently, the prosperity and resulting stress associated with capitalism caused the community's health to degenerate.

Money can also have a negative impact on a human being's attitude. When I was pursuing a master of commerce degree, my human resource professor surprised most of the class, including me, when he made a statement. To paraphrase his remark, "Money does not make employees happy in their jobs; instead, it is more likely to be the source of discontentment." In response to a challenge from one of the students, he explained, "Employees tend to compare their compensation to that of their co-workers, which can lead to unrest in the workplace."

Based on my personal experience, this theory is correct. Before I became self-employed, I worked for a company that would eventually become my competitor. On a particular Christmas occasion, the CEO of the company distributed bonuses to select staff members, and I was excluded. Almost immediately, the event became common knowledge throughout the firm. Although I wasn't expecting a bonus, I became irritated by the snub. It festered inside me, which prompted me to plan an exit from the company . . . on my terms. Over the course of the next few months, I recruited two key staff members, who were also working there and unhappy. It wasn't long before the three of us proudly announced we were leaving the firm to establish a competing business. As an aside, soon after we opened for business, when we were most vulnerable to fail, the CEO complained to the authorities about the name of our corporation. The Commonwealth of Virginia sent us a cease and desist order, and the issue went to court, which resulted in a compromise on the name. We were back in business, ready to compete ardently against the CEO and his company, which we did until our firm was sold.

Let's get back to the main topic. While it's true there can be negatives associated with wealth, a deficiency of wealth is undoubtedly discomforting. As previously stated, there is a direct correlation between an individual's prosperity and their sense of security, making wealth one of the factors in contentment. Imagine the anxiety, humiliation and unhappiness associated with having to accept welfare to obtain the bare necessities of life: shelter, food, clothing, medical services and so forth. A degree of wealth is not only necessary for survival, but also for peace of mind.

However, survival is one thing, avarice another. Catastrophic events aside, humans can survive very well for a long time without going over the top. Greed, the desire to attain a glut of wealth, is one of the seven deadly sins. And at least three other deadly sins – envy, lust and pride

– are often entwined in greed. Greed can also be the basis of felonies such as theft, fraud, robbery . . . or worse. Without appealing to the voracious nature of people in the form of unrealistic investment returns, Bernie Madoff would have been unable to lure a large number of sophisticated, astute individuals. And Madoff is just one example. Operating at levels well below that of Madoff, there have been and continue to be an overabundance of conmen that routinely use greed as a hook. They all rely on the fact that humans are seldom satisfied. This was unforgettably exampled by the amoral Gordon Gekko, portrayed by Michael Douglas in the movie *Wall Street*, who exclaimed, "Greed is good!" And, as in Gekko's case, it isn't uncommon for individuals with insatiable appetites for material goods to possess distorted senses of self-importance. Many of them use wealth as a means of self-glorification.

Some have hypothesized, "The reward is in the journey," meaning that people chasing and attaining riches receive more gratification from how they obtain fortunes than they do the resulting wealth. That may be true in some cases, but it is false in many others. Greedy individuals often measure themselves by the end result. Many aspire to possess more than others. Often, this type of individual is also disposed to resent anyone holding more than them. This is an exercise in futility. Just like the fastest gunslinger in Frontier American folklore, someone better is always lurking just around the corner.

There is also another negative characteristic of materialism that should be mentioned. It is difficult to be wealth-centered and people-centered at the same time. When an individual's choices are always driven to stockpile wealth, it usually comes at the expense of others. Hence, wealth-centered and people-centered ideologies tend to be mutually exclusive. Nonetheless, as previously stated, accumulating wealth is an inborn characteristic of humans. Thus, it requires strength and willpower to moderate the tendency to be *overly* attracted to wealth.

Those with the discipline to restrain themselves will avoid the dangers that overindulgence can bring.

One of the benefits of reaching the senior phase of life is that the instinct to accrue wealth for long-term survival diminishes; in the natural order of events, seniors have less time to live and don't need as much. Most people that continue to hoard late in life do so to protect their heirs' futures, not their own. Because this stimulus does not innately produce stress, seniors tend to be somewhat relaxed. Having acknowledged their destiny, they can more easily accept the highs and lows that life brings. This was adequately explained in a movie about a teenager and his grandfatherly mentor who were attempting to capture a wild mustang. After they toiled several days to erect and bait a corral, they waited patiently for the mustang. Almost immediately after the target was lured into the trap, it was spooked by another animal and it escaped. The old man accepted the exasperating misfortune calmly. The frustrated youngster looked at his mentor and remarked, "You just take things as they come." The old man explained, "When you've been around as long as I have, you'll get the hang of it."

Everyone's life has some degree of adversity. Those that roll with the emotional punches of hardships will be happier than those that take the full force of letdowns on the chin. Does this mean that humans shouldn't strive to predict and manage successful outcomes? Of course not. We should always strive for success. Nevertheless, it's important to be resilient when we don't achieve our goals.

To summarize, although a degree of wealth is necessary for peace of mind and happiness, it's best to reject greed as an ideology of life. Hence, I subscribe to the principle: *constrain the innate craving to possess too much wealth.*

CHAPTER 6
Work

Without applying a heavy dose of work, it is extremely difficult for us to accomplish anything important in life and it's effectively impossible for us to reach our full potential. For these reasons, the vast majority of us put forward a good effort during the adult phase of our lives. Regrettably, when we finally reach the senior phase, we begin to experience a natural decline in our energy and our ability to work. But should this transformation place us on a course of total unproductivity, especially in view of the fact that our longevity is on the upswing?

In America, there is certainly some pressure for seniors to remain productive longer; this is manifesting itself in Social Security. Specifically, the federal government has partially compensated for revenue shortfalls by extending the qualification age and penalizing for early withdrawals. This is actually a reasonable solution to ease the problem, but it appears that more will be needed.

However, not all of the government's tactics on Social Security are reasonable. For instance, some of our politicians have spouted claptrap that Social Security is a "government benefit" or an "entitlement." Unquestionably, Social Security is anything but a benefit or an entitlement. Most recipients, from the lowest to the highest social classes, paid into the fund, along with their employers, for decades. Disbursements to these individuals are simply the government returning some of the money it had seized, a toll it continues to exact on millions of working Americans. Instead of targeting individuals that endowed the program, the government should accept its responsibility for mismanaging the fund. Furthermore, politicians should stop using Social Security as a political weapon to threaten American citizens, such as Barack Obama did.

With that small digression on politics and politicians out of the way, let's get back to the topic of work.

IDLE HANDS

When I was a child, I attended a parochial elementary school and the teachers were Catholic nuns. They would often tell us: *"Idle hands are the devil's workshop."* Most of the students didn't fully appreciate the message at the time, but later in life we came to understand it very well. It was closer to the truth than not. If an individual's hands are idle, meaning they are being unproductive, there is a strong possibility that their mind is idle. And an idle mind is susceptible to an invading force called evil. Thus, "busy hands," or work, can be beneficial for an individual's mind, body and sprit. Conversely, "idle hands," or laziness, tends to damage an individual's mind, body and spirit. As an aside, while we're on the subject of hands, the nuns did something else that was noteworthy. To motivate us to be respectful and attentive, students that disobeyed classroom rules of order would receive a rap on the knuckles with a wood ruler.

DOES DNA MATTER?

At this point in time, most people are fully aware of the term DNA, the acronym for deoxyribonucleic acid, which is the carrier of genetic information in humans as well as other organisms on Earth. Most of us know little else about it. I've read a summary of one study that indicated certain DNA is associated with longevity. Although I'm unqualified to determine if this report is accurate or if my DNA actually controls my longevity, I can state one related fact with complete certainty: my father had prolonged longevity. He was able to work effectively as a bookkeeper until he was in his early nineties. And one of my uncles on my mother's side of the family also has prolonged longevity. The man is ninety-one years old and he looks like he's in his sixties; more importantly, he thinks and behaves like he's in his forties.

Attitude is important

Perhaps the blood running through my body predisposes me to be different than many retirees. Or perhaps the good health I currently enjoy in my mid-seventies has more to do with my philosophy on life. I can't answer that, but I can unequivocally state that a positive outlook does nothing to degrade an individual's health and/or their longevity. It was previously stated that life is not about breathing, but about having quality time for as long as possible. The adage "You are who you think you are" is entirely accurate. Individuals who believe they have accomplished everything they can have nothing to inspire them. And without a positive stimulus in life, it is my belief that the aging and dying process is likely to be accelerated. And I also believe the converse is true. Individuals that constantly look forward to achieving something are likely to improve the odds of having a longer, richer life.

To validate what attitude can accomplish, let me expound on the uncle I just mentioned and what his approach to life has done and continues to do for him. Considering his age, his state of mind and body, his active lifestyle, his instincts and the impediments he overcame to achieve success with his family and finances, he's one of the most remarkable people I've ever known. I've had many deep conversations with him, hoping to learn his secret to life. Eventually, I concluded that the differentiator between him and the majority of people his age is his boundless positive attitude, which gives him the energy and the enthusiasm to live. Refusing to knuckle down to the aging process, he rises each morning looking forward to the new day and what it has in store for him. He possesses an innate drive to remain an effective earner, and he has an appetite to enjoy the fruits of his labor. He has always found the right mix between working hard and playing hard – an ideal prescription for anyone – and he still does. When he was seventy-three, his first wife passed away. After a brief period of grief, he continued to mentor his four sons, three of whom were taking his land development business to new heights. Seven years later, at age eighty, he remarried. He and his second wife enjoy a very active lifestyle. He still wins at his favorite pastime, no limit Omaha poker. He didn't adopt his fast-paced régime in the hopes of defeating the grim reaper. Like with everything, his perspective on aging and death has been, and continues to be, pragmatic. He consistently professes his view on death, "I'm no kid. I know where I am in life. Death is approaching fast. I'm ready, but I'm not looking forward to it. When it's my time, I want to go quickly. I don't want to be a burden. If I could get my hands on one of those pills the Nazis bit, I'd keep it handy."

LEARNING TO WORK

I am a work-intensive person, which I attribute to my background. My parents were hard workers and showed me the way by their example and the way they raised me. If DNA is a determinant of longevity, perhaps it also affects work ethic. Whether it does or doesn't, my parents made certain that I got in touch with the meaning of work at the formative stage in my life, for which I am eternally grateful. At the age of thirteen, I began mowing and trimming lawns for fifty cents. I started out with a fully manual, reel lawn mower, which made the task of mowing much more difficult than it is today. Then I graduated to a rotary blade, gasoline engine mower, making the job easier. Later, at age fifteen, I stopped mowing lawns when my dad got me a summer job as a helper on a soft drink truck. The pay was eighteen dollars per week for fifty-five hours of hard manual labor. My duties were simple. After loading the truck each morning, I accompanied the driver on his daily route to see our customers, who were mostly smalltime retailers. When customers needed our merchandise, he wrote orders and collected payments, while I unloaded cases from the truck, hauled them into the stores and placed them where directed. My best friend became a handcart. At the end of the day, I rested very well.

To reinforce my parent's training, my high school and college, both of which were military, entrenched the principles of discipline and work ethic in every student, including me. During summers when I was not in school, I always kept a job. And after leaving the world of academia and until I retired, I was always employed. Twenty-five of those years, I was self-employed, which often demanded that I invest fifty-five+ hours per week at the firm, even when I served as its president and CEO for ten years.

Fortunately, God blessed me with excellent health, both physically and mentally, which allowed me to be productive. I consider the ability to work to be a privilege. Not everyone is so well off. Thus, work has always had a respected place in my life, and I hope it always will.

Work's Value

Many individuals work solely for the financial reward. This, undeniably, is a perfectly valid purpose. For the majority of my life, I did the same thing. The time I had on Earth was unknown and limited; consequently, time was precious to me, and I wanted to use most of what God gave me to protect my family's present and future.

In addition, I also derived an indirect benefit from work throughout my career, one that was intangible. It was always spiritually uplifting when I accomplished something, even small things that were practically insignificant. The emotional remuneration sometimes exceeded the monetary recompense.

These benefits apply to everyone healthy enough to work, even seniors. And should seniors choose to remain at least partially productive, there would likely be a positive impact on the economic problem that we currently face with Social Security and Medicare. Please note the use of "we" in lieu of "government." America's problems do not belong to elected politicians and government employees, but to its citizens. Still, even healthy seniors with the willingness to remain productive longer face barriers. This will be expanded upon in Chapter 11. Some seniors may be thinking, "I worked and paid taxes all of my life. Sure, I'm still healthy and I could contribute a little longer, but I didn't make the problem with Social Security. I have no intention of continuing to work, and I want what's coming to me." I have no reasonable argument against that line of thinking. Still, Social Security will remain a huge problem until it is fixed. *We the People* can't ignore the issue or hope that bureaucrats will advance a practical solution. Many of them appear too politically-fragmented and self-centered to fix anything.

Virtually every retired senior known to me has been a good producer, a contributor to civilization, the best part of what made America a great nation. And the majority of us have accumulated more wealth than necessary to enjoy a comfortable life until we die, leaving us with options about what to do with our surplus resources, both time and money. Should we siphon money from our nest eggs to enjoy leisurely pursuits or should we assume an intermediate position by devoting a portion of our time towards productive endeavors?

On the surface this would appear to have a simple answer. After all, senior citizens have earned the right to treat themselves. And there is certainly encouragement to play. We see an abundance of targeted advertising from retirement communities, tourist agencies and financial firms, which promote retirees living a long, carefree lifestyle, one without meaningful purpose or importance. The underlying theme of these ads is to encourage a lifestyle defined by pleasurable activities such as golf, travel, cruises and the like, conveying the subliminal message: you've earned it; have fun. In fact, some of these ads even hint at lowering the age expectancy for a laidback lifestyle by using actors, who appear to be younger than most seniors. The notion behind this seems to be in line with the fall of the Roman Empire, when indolence and decadence were factors in the destruction of a once prosperous society, obeying a rule of nature: too much of anything can be dangerous. In the case of the Romans, idleness was a significant contributor. Should we learn from history or should we ignore it?

This is not intended to oppose promotional campaigns designed to encourage saving and investing wisely. It is unquestionably appropriate and vitally important for all adults to save for the senior phase of life to sustain themselves in a reasonably good lifestyle. It's called survival, and it's harmful, even demeaning to be groveling for handouts from the government or from anyone, when one is capable of doing otherwise.

That said, what should seniors who exit the workforce in sound mental, physical and financial condition aspire to do with the rest of their lives? Should they squander all or part of their good fortune on lighthearted endeavors or should they pursue a reasonable balance between play and productivity?

PLAY'S VALUE

Life is most definitely not all about work. People need rest and relaxation. Even God saw it that way. One of His Ten Commandments prescribes working six days a week and reserving the seventh for the Sabbath Day, the Lord's Day. Man has, of course, taken liberties with this. Nowadays, very few Americans work six days a week, nor do most dedicate an entire day to their Creator.

And humans require more than just rest. We need some pleasurable activities in our lives. Not only do we think this is necessary, but so must God. Otherwise, He would not have set an example through His son Jesus Christ. The first miracle credited to Jesus was the Wedding at Cana, where Jesus transformed water into wine so the *festivities could continue*. In effect, this was a heavenly work to keep the party going.

Given that play has an important position in our lives, the question becomes how much time should be devoted to it.

Juggling work and play

As we advance through the phases of life and mature, our priorities for work and play change significantly. In the childhood phase, we generally have few responsibilities other than meeting the obligations of being a student, which predictably elevates play to a prominent place in our lives. But as we move through the adolescent phase into adulthood, we must increasingly adapt to the responsibilities of grownups, which entails work; this gradually reduces the amount of available time for pleasurable pursuits. Still, we never totally shed our childhood need to play. It becomes a matter of how much recreation, what activity and when. Most of us reserve a portion of our lives for leisurely pursuits with family, friends and business associates. These social occasions are always pleasant and relaxing elixirs for our spirits. There are significant differences between children and adult games, though. Adult games are usually more serious and the toys are much more expensive.

Eventually, we reach the senior phase of life and we lose many of the responsibilities we had in the adult phase. This gives seniors with good health and adequate financial means the freedom to make a conscientious choice on how to divide their resources between work and play.

Certainly play is gratifying, but so is work. In fact, work can exclude financial remuneration and still be satisfying. Generosity has its own form of reward. Not only is helping others spiritually uplifting, kindheartedness is looked upon favorably by our Creator. This is very important to Christians and can be a source of great contentment.

In the end, sound arguments can be made on both sides of the equation for work and play. Remembering that too much of anything can be dangerous, it is best to make a place for both and adopt the principle: *balance work and play.*

Chapter 7
Morality

It would not be shocking to learn that some readers will question the reason for a chapter devoted to *morality* in a book on aging, perhaps thinking the word is a misprint. After all, *mortality* is a more appropriate topic in the life of seniors, because they are closer to the end. In my view, there is no useful purpose to be served by probing the transient nature of life. We all understand that every human dies. The only variable with death is the circumstances surrounding it, the *how* and the *when* of it, which are essentially a matter of an individual's destiny. Why waste time analyzing something that we must accept? And for those preparing to make the transition from their temporal bodies, there are certainly available and willing specialists that can help individuals manage the process.

This book is about improving the progression of aging, and there is a perfectly valid reason to incorporate a chapter on morality. An individual's righteousness affects reaching bliss after death, which should be the goal of every Christian and others believing in Eternal Life, and it can also enhance our sense of self-gratification while we're alive. And for those possessing a conscience, ethic-centered behavior is a variable, over which well-intended individuals can exercise a modicum of control.

HUMAN BEHAVIOR

The right and wrong of a human action is a resultant of the underlying motive behind the act and the consequences of it. For instance, let's briefly examine the moral act of sexual intercourse between willing men and women. The urge to engage in sex is a built-in characteristic of human beings. The purpose of mating is to perpetuate life, and the deed is part of our instinct for survival. The sensation attached to orgasms is euphoric, which disposes mating partners to become sexually aroused and to engage in intercourse. When the act is performed properly, although the feeling is fleeting, the fulfillment that loving partners can derive from surrendering themselves for the purpose of each other's pleasure is second to none.

However, not everyone is aroused for the right reason nor does everyone use sex as it was intended to be practiced. Rapists, who are depraved monsters personifying evil, use sex as a tool to satiate their warped fantasies or to impose their will upon coerced humans or both. To them, sex is a totally self-serving, violent act. They derive pleasure from the victim's suffering. After rapists satisfy their malevolent urges, many of the victims lucky enough to survive such attacks are left with deep emotional scars.

The distinction is clear. Sex can be used either for good or for evil.

LAWS AND HUMAN BEHAVIOR

For those of us that honor Jesus Christ and His Father, the Ten Commandments are heavenly laws that set a standard of human behavior on Earth. The punishment attached to disobeying these laws, or sins against God, is somewhat obscure. Christians believe that unrepentant sinners will face judgement in the Afterlife. However, not everyone is a Christian. And even those that are Christians may not subscribe to this faith-based concept. Thus, not everyone abides by God's standard of behavior.

Not only did God create laws to guide human behavior, so did society. Disobeying society's laws have prescribed, tangible consequences. Nonetheless, not everyone obeys man's laws either.

To complicate matters, the right and wrong of a specific act isn't always easy to judge. Take murder, for instance. Humans killing humans, which by rule is a violation of man's laws and God's laws, is not always wrong. Sometimes humans kill other humans for entirely justifiable, righteous reasons. Unusual circumstances can leave no reasonable alternative, such as killings motivated by self-defense or to prevent wide-scale murder. Few would argue that using any means necessary, including killing, to prevent a home invader from enacting violence on innocent victims, is wrong. Likewise, the same holds true when it comes to exterminating terrorists, whose business is to engage in appalling crimes against masses of humanity. Aside from disciples of Osama bin Laden, we would find few humans that believe eradicating him was wrong. His execution ridded the world of a savage, cowardly mass-murderer, who was disposed to continue until he was stopped. Most people believe that destroying him was right and that it did not happen soon enough.

It is not uncommon for circumstantial variables surrounding individual situations, which aren't specified in the general nature of either the laws of God or the laws of man or both, to become key determinants in establishing the right and wrong of human behavior; these often fall into an unclear area, one that requires judgment, a determination of the human conscience made by applying logic and one's sense of morality.

Morality and conscience

Most, but certainly not all, humans are born with a sense of self-awareness known as the human conscience that allows them to distinguish between right and wrong. Those with a conscience can comprehend the implications of their conduct and intent. Behavior can be influenced by this intellectual regulator; and it can also be governed by the natural tendency of humans to be self-serving, a derivative of the innate instinct to survive. Just how far an individual will go to help themselves at the expense of others is a matter of how they perceive the consequences of their acts and how much discipline they can exercise to control themselves. In effect, humans serve as their own judge and jury on the matter of right and wrong. What is considered to be right by one person, may be considered to be wrong by another, and vice-versa. And to others, the identical situation may fall into a middle-ground, an unclear area, which is neither right nor wrong.

Christians often refer to general guidelines contained in the New Testament of the Bible to help them with decisions. One of these guidelines is found in Luke 6:31, "And as ye would that men should do to you, do ye also to them likewise." In essence, this conveys the concept that we should behave in a manner that is not harmful to others, because we would not wish others to harm us. And because self-serving behavior can be harmful to others, we should consider its effect.

Let's examine this concept more closely using the line graph below titled Morals.

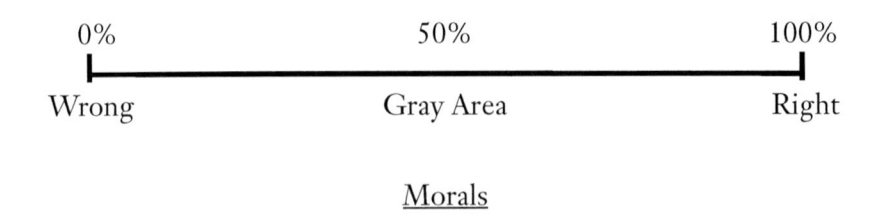

```
0%                    50%                   100%
|——————————————————————————————————————————|
Wrong              Gray Area                Right
```

<u>Morals</u>

Individuals that consistently and knowingly do what is best for them irrespective of the consequence to others would fall to the extreme left, which is defined by the term Wrong. Explaining this in a different way, completely self-serving behavior can be harmful to others; thus, it is wrong because it defies the basic idea established in Luke 6:31. On the opposite end of the spectrum, individuals that consistently reject self-serving behavior in order to do what it best for others would fall to the extreme right, which is defined by the term Right. Other than rare exceptions like Mother Teresa, humans don't fall into this category. Unquestionably, the majority of people fall somewhere between Right and Wrong, or in the Gray Area.

The next graph, which is titled Selflessness, depicts the parallel between selflessness and right and wrong.

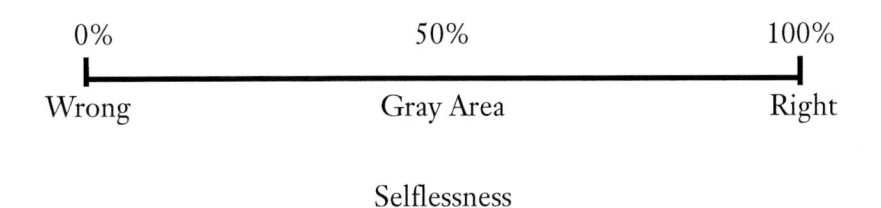

```
0%                      50%                    100%
|────────────────────────┼────────────────────────|
Wrong                 Gray Area                 Right
```

<u>Selflessness</u>

Individuals, whose behavior is 0% selfless, would fail the standard in Luke 6:31; therefore, it would be Wrong. On the opposite end of the spectrum, individuals who are consistently 100% selfless would be categorized as Right; again, humans exhibiting that behavior are rare. Consequently, most humans fall in the Gray Area somewhere between 0% selfless or Wrong and 100% selfless or Right.

The point of these simple graphics is to demonstrate that morals, a powerful, underlying force in human behavior, can vary significantly, depending on the nature and the judgement of individuals. The human conscience is the resource for answers to disconcerting questions that often arise when making important decisions. Should I do what is best for me, disregarding the consequence to others, or should I sacrifice? Or should I take a positon in the middle?

These choices arise frequently. Take charitable contributions, for instance. Should those with significant monetary resources donate ten dollars a week to their church, a hundred or a thousand? Should they donate five dollars to help needy individuals, five hundred or five thousand? How much is reasonable? This becomes a matter of judgement, and the human conscience is the decider, the reference that yields an answer.

This parallels a concept on greed I mentioned previously: the ideals of being wealth-centered and people-centered tend to be mutually exclusive. Expressing this theory differently, a voracious appetite for wealth is selfish if and when sating our urges comes at the expense of others, which is highly likely.

As an aside, I prefer associating with people that lean somewhere to the right on the Selflessness graph, towards the selfless end. People disposed in that direction tend to be loyal when times get tough. And, sooner or later, times always get tough. With regard to those inclined towards the 0% selfless end on the far left, they tend to be fair-weathered friends. At the first sign of trouble, they are prone to do whatever is necessary to serve their best interest at the expense of anyone and everyone.

Should we expect people to be 100% selfless? Absolutely not. This would contradict our survival instinct and subject us to extreme hardships in life. For this reason, we cannot totally rely upon the good nature of our fellow man for our survival.

That said, how should we behave? Should we be selfish or selfless? In addition to Luke 6:31, we can find a clue in this passage from Mark 12:31 found in the New Testament: "And the second is like, namely this, *Thou shalt love thy neighbor as thyself.* There is none other commandment greater than these." In essence, this passage sets in stone the principle of compromise. Although it recognizes that humans should love their neighbors, it allows that we can love ourselves.

Human behavior that falls in the gray area somewhere between 0% selfless or Wrong and 100% selfless or Right on the Selflessness graph, a reasonable balance between the extremes, would meet the biblical criteria. Although an *acceptable* degree of self-serving behavior isn't wrong, an *unacceptable* degree of it is. The regulator for what is acceptable or unacceptable, what is right or wrong, what is moral or immoral, is that imperceptible part of us called the human conscience. And, for those that possess a conscience, acts of sacrifice can be extremely rewarding, uplifting experiences. Consequently, we should strive to live by the principle: *balance self-serving behavior with sacrifice.*

Chapter 8
Spirituality

Many prefer to avoid discussing politics and religion. I generally agree with that attitude, because these topics tend to provoke controversy, which can rapidly evolve into confrontation or worse. Nevertheless, in my view, it is impossible to present ideologies on life, and particularly on aging, without including a little information on politics and an extensive amount on spirituality. In fact, because of spirituality's importance, this chapter is devoted entirely to it. Whenever spirituality is on the table, Eternal Life and God are the primary concepts to examine.

Eternal Life and God

Heaven, where the throne of God is promised to exist, is said to be an unequalled, timeless place of bliss. Humans are mortal and our bodies are designed to be short-lived. We can feel our spirit, but we can't see it. Yet, it is our spirit that is said to be able to transcend death, and its fate is in the hands of an unseen, immortal God. The pragmatic part of the human brain makes the theory of God difficult to rationalize, comprehend and accept.

And likewise, the concept of everlasting bliss is challenging to rationalize, comprehend and accept. Although we can reach blissful states from time to time, the sensations never last very long. It is almost as if those momentary encounters are intended to tease us, make us contemplate the potential of endless bliss in Eternal Life. There is no doubt that vague, baffling concept called Eternal Life is riddled with mystery and controversy. In my view, a clandestine plot is ideal for an entertaining novel or a movie, but mystery is far from perfect for matters concerning real life and death. Most people would like to be confident in the truth about Eternal Life. I certainly wanted to be assured that it existed. I wanted to remove the murky cloud that concealed the unknown. I wanted to know whether or not Heaven was real. And if it was real, what was it like? Did I actually break through that veil and find the secret? I hope so, and I went all-in and risked what's left of my life and my soul, trusting that I did.

Later, you will discover that I have always had faith in the existence of God. Even though I have not seen Him, He is real. You see, I can't reasonably explain life without Him, and neither can anyone else I know. The preciseness of life's order coupled with the variety and the intricate design of the innumerable lifeforms roaming Earth are unfathomable without the presence and work of a Creator possessing abilities far greater than man. For those that disagree, ask yourself a simple question: could an assemblage of the most elite, most brilliant scientists that inhabit our world create an ant or a mouse or a dolphin or an oak tree or any life-form of their choice from nothing? If they can do it, the world is waiting to watch the show.

Although I had accepted God, Eternal Life was a completely different matter. To be perfectly candid, during my life I equivocated on it many times. Like almost every human that has ever drawn a breath, I tend to believe what I see and I have never seen Heaven. Sure, there are a few people that have proclaimed to have seen it, but in my mind these declarations do not necessarily have to be true . . . nor do they necessarily have to be false.

That said, I have also never seen Jesus Christ or Napoleon Bonaparte or Abraham Lincoln or Leonardo Da Vinci or Albert Einstein, to name just a few, but I believe they all walked the planet Earth. Similarly, I was not an eyewitness to the Battle of the Bulge or the Black Death or the Niña, the Pinta and the Santa Maria crossing the Atlantic Ocean, but I believe those events did occur. Why? Because history has carefully documented the facts, giving me little choice but to accept them as having been real.

Likewise, Heaven and Eternal Life must exist. After all, the New Testament of the Bible, a historical source like any other, documented Jesus Christ referencing the existence of Eternal Life. And to prove His point, after His crucifixion and death, He resurrected from the dead and appeared. When He did, He made a powerful commitment to believers, which is recorded in John 20:29, the account of Jesus addressing His doubting disciple Thomas upon His return, "Jesus saith unto him, Thomas, because thou hast seen me, thou hast believed: *blessed are they that have not seen, and yet have believed.*" Who am I to cast uncertainty on what Jesus Christ said and did? And the life, death and resurrection of Christ is not the only reason to believe in Eternal Life. Even without any biblical evidence to validate the concept, it would be unreasonable to deduce that life after death does not exist. Without the reality of God and the promise of Eternal Life, there is simply no logical explanation for our existence and the stern test that we must pass. Christians subscribe to the belief that Jesus Christ was on the Earth to give us a chance to join Him in Eternal Life. Simply stated, Jesus gave us hope; following His way of life bridges the chasm between life and death. Without the hope of perpetuity in Eternal Life, the notion of life is mind-bending and its challenges unbearable. Hence, being assured of an unimaginable place where human souls delight in euphoria brings peace of mind to Christians.

Does every declared Christian believe in Eternal Life and do they follow Christ's recipe to get there? I think the answer is no. Let me explain why I hold this belief. As some Christians move through the stages of life, they clearly demonstrate their intent to hold onto life and its trappings forever. They resist the idea of dying. In my view, this is inconsistent with the promise of Christ. Any Christian that truly believes in Christ's promise and emulates His way should look forward to death. In the sanctuary of Eternal Life, we exchange the trinkets that life offers, along with life's pain and suffering, for endless bliss.

Some people have claimed they visited Heaven. I'm likely not alone in wanting to believe that other mortals have seen it. Unfortunately, most humans, including me, have an inborn distrust of anything we haven't experienced. Because I haven't been in Heaven, it's easy to have reservations about the accuracy of such statements. Does this mean such assertions are untrue? Of course, not. Nonetheless, the best way – and possibly the only way – for most of us to accept the existence of Heaven and Eternal Life is to possess faith. Those aspiring to believe in the Afterlife wholeheartedly, yet who have lingering doubts, will always be wanting unless they have conviction in Jesus Christ. Trust is everything, and especially with a concept as deep as life after death.

My favorite priest of all time, a truly wonderful mentor and Benedictine Monk who is now deceased, once shared this quote from one of his dying parishioners, "Faith is what you have, when you don't have anything else." That about sums it up, doesn't it?

As for me, I can honestly say that I'm not afraid of death. Even though I haven't seen Heaven, I'll go along with Jesus Christ and His promise that it exists. And, most particularly, I refuse to take any risk that it does exist and that I didn't do enough to get there.

Religion

I was baptized and raised as a Christian, and more specifically as a Roman Catholic. Primarily due to my dad, as a child I was exposed to almost everything the Roman Catholic Church had to offer. My religious training intensified in parochial elementary school, where my friends and I studied the fundamentals of Catholicism in addition to a normal educational curriculum. I received the sacraments of Reconciliation, Eucharist and Confirmation, and I served as an altar boy for daily and Sunday masses. In order to serve God and my church, I got an early start on those days, a habit that has remained with me for the entirety of my life. At the time I served as an altar boy, I thought it was a privilege, and I still do, sixty+ years later. After finishing elementary school, I attended a Christocentric, all-boys, military high school. Most of the instructors were Benedictine Monks, and they augmented our academic training with religion. We were also given a heavy dose of discipline, something that has served me well over my entire life.

While I was going through the childhood and adolescent phases of life, I was unaware that my dad, prior to marrying my mom, had studied to be a Catholic priest. Later, I became informed that he was removed from the priesthood program because of a question relating to the legality of his parents' marriage. Although his removal from the program paved the way for my eventual existence, that decision denied the church the services of a truly righteous man, who would have been a terrific representative of God. After dad passed away, I discovered a handwritten paper authored by him. It outlined his enduring love for God and the Catholic Church. I already knew his relationship with God and the church was truly special. Following Christ's example, he lived a peaceful, humble life, which was focused on prayer and service to his fellow man: family, friends, others in need. And his memoir taught me something that I didn't know. He had been an acolyte, an assistant in liturgical service, for eighty years. That's not a misprint; he served for *eighty* years. Although my dad was a staunch Catholic, he respected and was open to the views of others, including different religious ideals.

I CHANGED

The strong religious foundation, which was built during my childhood and adolescent phases, began to weaken when I entered the adult phase of my life. Looking back on it now, I can see some of the factors that contributed to it. First and foremost, my ego began to assert itself. I wanted to stake my own turf in life, to be my own man. Perhaps I became a bit rebellious, and I was looking for excuses to reject my faith.

And it was easy to find faults with my religion. The use of Latin in the mass bothered me; the vast majority of parishioners, including me, didn't understand the language, so there was a major disconnect in following the rites. As an aside, English eventually replaced Latin throughout most of the United States, and this change greatly improved the experience of attending services.

I also disagreed with the Sacrament of Reconciliation (Confession). To obtain forgiveness for my sins, I didn't understand why it was necessary to humble myself by exposing my flaws to a priest. After all, they were human, too. I believed it was better to ask God directly for forgiveness and to reconcile with those adversely affected by my wrongdoings. Regrettably, I didn't always follow my method, though.

After enrolling in college, I shifted further away from my faith. Most of my energy was focused on academics, which I prioritized over everything. Only occasionally would I make an appearance at the local church. Later, after I entered the military, I continued to have little interest in my religion. Even after I was assigned to Vietnam, rarely did I attend mass. Certainly, my combat engineer duties didn't put me in as much danger as those in the infantry, but I was still at risk of being severely injured or killed. I should have wanted to stay on excellent terms with God, but I often shunned it.

After I was married, the weakening of my religious foundation continued. I was upset by a flood of crimes that had been perpetrated by rogue clergymen, some of whom were Catholic priests. Certainly, the cases were exceptions, not the standard. Most clergymen lived moral lives. Nevertheless, because the ranks of clergymen had been infiltrated by evil, I believed that God would undoubtedly forgive anyone like me for doubting the sanctity of religious groups.

Then there was Catholicism's stance on contraception. My wife and I practiced birth control, and we didn't want to be censured for managing the number of offspring we produced and supported.

I also rejected associating with those attending church that in my judgment were not living by Christ's standards. After leaving church, they tended to revert back to their egocentric endeavors and throw out sayings like, "Life is hard, but it's fair" or "I'm only doing to them what they would do to me." In essence, taking advantage of others is acceptable.

There was something else about the Catholic Church that disturbed me. It projected an image of extravagance. I could not link the needy, humble personality of Jesus Christ with the decadence that surrounded my religion. After touring monuments such as the Sistine Chapel in Rome and the Santa Maria del Fiore in Florence, they elicited a swarm of questions: How much did these wonders cost? Who paid for them? How were they constructed? How many people died erecting them? Does the modern world have the talent to replicate them at any price? Considering the level of poverty that still existed in the world, the excess was difficult to accept.

And then there was another reason to shun religion, an even stronger reason. Throughout the history of the world, religious and political dogma had been the underpinning of horrible crimes against humanity. Religion had spawned malicious individuals that were obsessed with persecution in the name of God. An example is the Crusades, military campaigns sanctioned by various popes. Another is the Spanish Inquisition. And in the modern world, radical Muslim groups use terrorism to kill, maim and destroy shamelessly, indiscriminately. And, while we're on the subject of terrorism, this unique form of social dysfunction and hostility needs to be summarily exterminated from every obscure corner of the world. Humanity has no place for individuals or groups that remorselessly brutalize others. These errand boys of death and evil operate under the subterfuge of holy crusaders. Conceptually, the notion of carnage being acceptable to any deity is a contradiction of the highest order; it defies the imagination, at least to people that adore a benevolent God. Christians certainly don't understand it. We're taught to be tolerant of others, despite our differences.

With that digression out of the way, the case I had built against religion had been compelling enough to assuage my conscience; I was perfectly comfortable not to practice my faith. Did adopting such a philosophy mean that I didn't not believe in God? Certainly not. I believed in His existence. However, I also held that religion and God were not necessarily mutually inclusive. Hence, in a free society like America's, Christians like me could revere God and Jesus Christ with or without the help of any group. After all, we have a conscience, the one He gave us, which is our guide on matters of right and wrong. Whenever I committed a wrongful act, my conscience reeled me in; it immediately triggered a remorseful reaction and the desire to atone.

Notwithstanding all these reasons, as I grew older and wiser, I began to have misgivings about my stance on religion and I wrestled with my conscience. Certainly the Catholic Church had collected its share of blemishes over its lengthy history. However, when I thought about my religion fairly instead of looking at its record through the selective lens of a member in poor standing, I realized that a few chinks in its armor were entirely reasonable. Churches are comprised of people . . . lots and lots of people. The seeds of evil – mendacity, transgressions and so forth – that occasionally sprout from religious entities are planted by wicked individuals that misrepresent the position of the church. Perhaps I was wrong to demand too much of my faith. And perhaps I was wrong to expect every Christian clergyman to not only talk Jesus's talk, but to walk His walk. That is an onerous expectation to mandate, especially given the large number of men that had populated the ranks of Catholic priesthood over the centuries. Most of all, who was I to judge anybody, and who was I to dictate such tough terms? I was just another sinner who was going through the motions in life, hoping to survive and to enjoy themselves as best they could.

I certainly had good reasons to give religion another look. I wanted to reach Eternal Life and I wanted to attain happiness on a more consistent basis on Earth. Spending some time with God each week could help accomplish both. The habit could provide regular maintenance on my soul and constantly reinforce hope, which is an anti-anxiety elixir. These considerations caused me to relook at religion from a fresh perspective. When I did, I was forced to admit that I had been wrong. Over the decades, I had allowed my self-absorbed nature to drive my beliefs and actions, including my position on religion. In my mind, I had considered myself to be a vital cog in the world, and I didn't need anyone or anything. Because an individual has reached adulthood does not mean they have maturity or wisdom. In fact, many adults I have observed over the years, including myself, have problems in these areas. You see, everyone is burdened by that human weakness called *ego*, which has the potential to be extremely harmful. It can remove all or part of a human's foundation. And in my case, my ego had been instrumental in me disavowing religion.

When I admitted my mistake, I began to work on overcoming my weaknesses, starting with dampening my sense of self. Whenever my unabashed ego begins to raise its ugly head, I pause to remind it, "Hold on, Big Boy! Make yourself scarce. You're at cross-purposes with your master. I'm on my way to bliss. You, on the other hand, may be on the way straight to hell."

At this final stage of my life, I have been able to see things more clearly than ever before. My brain is more mature and it's wiser; it told me to avoid sin, especially now that I am approaching the end of my life. It also told me to give religion an opportunity to help me reach my goals, which is why I adopted the principle: *love God and give religion its proper place.*

Chapter 9

Fitness

Similar to manmade machines, even that remarkable creation of God we call the human body can be abused. It has design limitations, which if ignored will lead to premature failure. In addition to the potential of being harmed by mistreatment, these unrivaled mechanisms comprised of organic matter can get out of adjustment. To keep them running in tiptop condition, they require the proper fuel and a regimen of appropriate upkeep. Ignoring the operating necessities can lead to poor performance or worse.

In developed countries like the United States, the vast majority of individuals take care of their medical needs. We are proactive in scheduling regular checkups, and should we encounter health problems between visits, we usually seek professional medical services right away, in particular whenever we suffer a health emergency.

However, there is much more to keeping the human body in good condition than trips to doctor's offices and hospitals. In addition to obtaining medical services, we need to perform regular maintenance on our bodies to keep them working effectively and efficiently. This is concentrated in three general categories: (1) consuming appropriate nourishment in sensible quantities, (2) exercising our brains and (3) exercising our bodies. In the context of this book, these are referred to as the Fitness Trio. The responsibility to manage the Fitness Trio inevitably falls to the affected individual, the owner of the body. We can either do the job properly or ignore it.

In the corporate world, businesses have been likened to a three-legged stool with marketing, finance and production each being a leg. When one leg is weak, the stool will become unstable. And should one leg break, the stool will collapse. There is a parallel between the three-legged stool of the corporate world and the Fitness Trio of the human body. Each of the three maintenance items – the legs that keep the human body upright – must be looked after and working well to optimize performance. If one leg is disregarded for an extended period, the body will likely become unsteady. If one leg is ignored completely, the body will deteriorate and will eventually fail.

Learning the Fitness Trio

When I began high school, I was exposed to the concept of staying physically and mentally fit. Of course, every student was challenged to exercise their mind in the classroom, but we were also required to exercise our bodies, even those not talented enough to participate on the school's sports teams. In gym class we did push-ups, sit-ups, jumping-jacks and so forth. In addition, we competed in volleyball, basketball, boxing, gymnastics and other games. These regular workouts helped to develop our bodies in a positive way. And the physical training improved my level of alertness and mental effectiveness, which helped me perform better in the classroom. In the senior phase of my life, I learned the scientific reason why the physical training had boosted my state of mind. Consistent physical exercise induces neurobiological benefits such as improvement in certain cognitive functions, improved stress coping and enhanced memory. Vigorous exercise can release chemicals called endorphins in the bloodstream, which are produced in the central nervous system and the pituitary gland; these trigger a positive feeling in the body and an energized outlook. And I also believe that mental fitness is conducive to physical fitness. When our minds are thriving, we are confident about ourselves; this state tends to produce energy, which can be released through work and physical exercise.

As for learning about the third leg, proper nourishment, my parents put me on the right path and they kept me on it until I flew their nest. They exhibited discipline in everything they did, including eating and drinking. Overeating at the table was impossible; my mom, who was a terrific cook, served reasonable portions of healthy, well-balanced meals that were absent of a lot of sugar or fat or overdoses of salt. She would consume even smaller helpings than she distributed to dad and me. If she was hungry between meals, she would nibble on a few crackers or a slice of cheese or consume a glass of milk. Thus, through my parents' example, I became grounded in sensible eating habits.

After I married, I learned that my wife – a superior cook in her own right – was also accustomed to small portions of food, only for a different reason. She was one of six children, and the household did not have a surplus of money. The family had enough to eat, but not an abundance of food. Consequently, from the very start of our marriage, my wife and I were in sync with regard to eating and drinking moderately. Our breakfast and dinner meals were frequently prepared at home, where we could control what we ate and when. Even now in the senior phases of our lives, although my wife and I can afford to dine out more often, we only do it a few times a week. We favor home-cooked meals because we can better control our nutrition and our dining experience in the quiet of our home.

Neither my wife nor I are nutritionists; we have never devoted an inordinate amount of time to analyze and/or restrict and/or measure our intake of calories, carbohydrates and the like. Yes, we have both tried diets in the past, but we have always reverted back to our core eating habits, which consists of a few simple basics. I was recently asked what I eat. For those that may be interested, I follow a guideline defined mostly by common sense. Generally, I avoid food products containing significant amounts of salt or saturated fat. Whenever my wife or I fry something, we use extra-virgin olive oil or vegetable oil. I never ingest soft drinks and usually consume forty to sixty ounces of water each day. As for alcoholic beverages, which I consume *moderately* in social settings, I prefer red wine or single malt Scotch Whiskey. In hot, humid weather, beer is my choice. When my schedule permits, I avoid solid food after 7:30 p.m., which usually allows several hours to digest nutrients before I retire for the night.

As for meals prepared at home, breakfast typically consists of apple juice, a cup of black coffee and a small bowl of dry bran cereal with a banana or a multigrain muffin with honey. I don't always eat lunch, but when I do it's something light such as a small bowl of homemade soup or cheese and crackers or homemade chicken salad or a multigrain muffin with peanut butter. Dinner is the main meal. Two or three times a week, it consists of a serving of meat – mostly chicken or pork – with a starch and/or a vegetable. Occasionally, a good hamburger or a steak or a bowl of Brunswick stew or my wife's tri-meat sauce over pasta finds its way on our table. On the other days, the menu is usually rice and beans or fish and a starch or pasta with veggies sautéed in a seasoned red (tomato based) or white (olive oil based) sauce or a homemade panini, plus a dessert. Yes, a *moderate* amount of bread and dessert is on the menu. If I get hungry between meals, I snack on a small portion of nuts or a few wedges of cheese or a piece of fruit.

Like many others that are attentive to their health, my wife and I monitor our weight, our cholesterol level and our blood pressure on a routine basis; we follow our doctor's advice with all three. If and when we gain a few pounds, we usually make a slight adjustment to our diet, such as reducing or abstaining from bread and desserts.

Mental exercise

As for keeping mentally fit, during my engineering career, which covered the majority of the adult phase of my life, my mind never lacked for exercise. After I became a husband and father, I was the family's primary provider. I had to constantly use my brain, hoping to be successful in the most important competition life has to offer: survival. When I was on the job, I had to be intellectually sharp, prepared to do my best to earn a living for my family. And I spent a vast number of hours on the job because there was no option. In fact, my brain got so much exercise that it would sometimes become overworked. Therefore, this leg of the Fitness Trio was never in danger of being overlooked. When the time for retirement arrived, I brought with me a mind that was in excellent condition. But I also knew that it would not remain sharp very long unless I found something to keep it honed.

A lifestyle of exercise & sports

I always considered the ability to work to be an honor, and I hold the same attitude with regard to physical exercise. Not everyone is as blessed physically as I was and still am; some people, through no fault of their own, are forced to go through life with handicaps that severely restrict or prevent them from exercising their minds and/or their bodies. And quite often they can do little or nothing to overturn their misfortune.

During most of the adult phase of my life, I relied on sports as the primary vehicle to exercise my body. Even as a youngster, I enjoyed participating in sports. For me sports weren't just fun. They gave me a good outlet for my energy and my competitive nature and a way to keep my body in shape. However, I was never blessed with a lot of natural athletic ability. This became abundantly clear when I tried out for teams and individual sports in high school, where my athletic flaws became quickly exposed.

When I became an adult, I still wanted to engage in sports, and so did many of my male associates and friends; most of them participated in something. During that era in the American culture, softball, handball, swimming, racquetball, golf, bowling, cycling, jogging and tennis were popular adult recreational activities. I knew it was important to select one or two of them, and I did.

In the early stages of my adulthood, when my children were small, I became interested in golf. I enjoyed the immense challenge of the game. It was me against me, and it took a tremendous amount of skill to consistently execute shots well. I quickly became an ardent fan of Jack Nicklaus, who I still consider to be among the best *sportsmen*, if not the greatest, to ever live. This sports legend was a fierce competitor who knew how to win and how to lose with dignity. Unfortunately, golf was an expensive pursuit with regard to time and money, and I was in short supply of both. The game also provided little of something else I craved: good physical workouts. Most golfers were no longer walking the courses; they were using motorized golf carts, and when I played, so did I.

In order to get physical exercise, I took up handball. Not only was the sport inexpensive, the workouts were terrific and they took very little time. By the middle of a game, I would be soaked with perspiration. At the local YMCA where I competed, players were categorized A, B or C level. Although I was getting a lot of exercise, I never rose above B level, which was similar to the average athletic talent I had displayed in other sports. When I was approaching thirty years of age, my body began to manifest signs that it was time to change sports. My shot-making ability was deteriorating slightly and my proneness to injury was increasing marginally. At some point, when I had lost enough points and absorbed enough bruises and dislocated fingers, I decided to make a change.

Tennis was a game that I had learned as a teenager. It was on the rise, and it was inexpensive with regard to time and money. Even more importantly, it was possible to make tennis a family affair, which our family did. My wife took up the game and so did our two daughters. They all became good players. Depending on the United States Tennis Association rater and the year I was rated, I competed at 3.5 or 4.0 levels, which was about the same as other sports I had tried. Nevertheless, I was getting a lot of exercise and making new friends, some of whom are still in my inner-circle today. On the days I wasn't working late or travelling, after dinner our family would steadfastly go to the local swim and racquet center. We always found matches there, which gave me an outlet to release the stress of the workday.

As though that wasn't enough, I was also jogging a few miles, three days a week. After several years of running, I began to experience knee, ankle, hip and low back problems. I tried better shoes, but they only provided marginal relief from the pounding. I was left with no choice. I had to stop jogging.

With respect to tennis, by the time I reached fifty, I had lost the ability to consistently reach shots on time, and I could no longer execute them as well as I had in the past. Dissatisfied with my performance, it was time to move to something else.

During those tennis years, I had managed to play about fifteen rounds of golf per year, many of which were business related. My handicap at the time was about twenty. After giving up tennis, I was at a point in my life where I had more time and money available; therefore, I gradually increased the number of rounds of golf. I found the game much harder than tennis, which only penalized players a single point for each mishit. In golf, competitors had to play their errant shots, which often resulted in a more severe penalty than a single stroke. Eventually, I lowered my handicap to the mid-teens. I had become a decent player, similar to what I had always done in other sports.

Until I gave up tennis at the age of fifty, I had done a reasonably good job of taking care of each leg in the Fitness Trio. That's when things began to fall apart. All I was doing was playing golf. As I mentioned earlier, I was using motorized golf carts to make my way around the courses. Hence, I was not getting the physical exercise I needed or wanted, and problems related to the lack of exercise began to manifest themselves.

Fortunately, thanks to my eating habits, my weight was still under control. In my early sixties, I only weighed about ten pounds more than the day I graduated from high school.

My physical condition was another matter. The muscles in my arms were getting weak. My midriff was getting bigger as a result of lack of exercise and weak abdominal muscles, and it was sagging noticeably thanks to Sir Isaac Newton's law of universal gravitation. And I was suffering from frequent low back problems, a derivative of my feeble core muscles. I would also get out of breath easily, an indication that my cardiovascular system was not performing as well as it should. I did not feel good, and my lack of physical conditioning was beginning to impact me mentally. In order to prevent further deterioration, it would be necessary to reenergize the Fitness Trio principle that I had followed most of my life: *exercise physically and mentally, while nourishing the body properly.*

Chapter 10
Legacy

From the moment humans are born, we begin the process of dying. Most of us don't spend a lot of time thinking about our mortality until we learn of a deadly condition or we reach the senior phase of our lives. When we are approaching the end, we begin to prepare for departing Earth. It is then that we are inclined to look back and evaluate our lives, including our failures and our achievements. As we go through life, most of us hoard assets, tangible goods of value. Unable to take these goods with us, we typically bequeath everything we own to individual(s) and/or organization(s) that we wish to help. The sum total of such gifts is commonly referred to as *legacy*.

Although this term has gained popularity among adults, and particularly among seniors, I do not recall hearing it mentioned very often until the latter part of the 20th Century. I don't know why this happened. Perhaps I became more aware of my legacy as a senior because of my closer proximity to death or because my station in life had improved. Or perhaps it was related to the unparalleled prosperity of a global economy that had been artificially propped up by debt. One thing is undoubtedly true. Materialism had reached a new plateau, one that was higher than it had ever been. Many seniors had amassed wealth; they owned property,

IRAs, stocks, bonds, precious metals, pension funds, bank accounts and the like.

Did prosperity change the way people thought of themselves? Maybe. For those able to bestow a substantial portfolio to their heirs, perhaps it served as testament to the excellent job they had done going through life. Pride is an interesting characteristic that can be associated with the monetary value of legacies, and it can elicit an indirect arms race of sorts. I have heard several seniors make comments like, "My net worth is (fill in the blank)" or "I'm leaving a trust fund of (fill in the blank)" or "I've already given my kids or grandkids (fill in the blank)." Some were on obvious fishing expeditions, hoping to glean information for the purpose of comparison. Their monetary status was a barometer to measure the value of their lives against others. Did they believe it defined who they were? Maybe. And why not? It is certainly reasonable for people, especially seniors, to value wealth so highly. After all, they worked most of their lives to earn as much as they could, and many had stockpiled a large surplus.

However, using that yardstick alone to measure the value of one's life is far from a fair assessment. Without demeaning the importance of money and property, the wealth that anyone accumulates and leaves in an estate is only a small fraction of who they are or who they will be perceived to be after they're dead, even to their heirs. Shortly after beneficiaries receive whatever is bequeathed, they typically make plans to use it, with little regard for the benefactor or the sacrifices made. It's quite natural for humans to discount the value of anything obtained without hard work. This is one reason why legacies should encompass more than tangible assets.

The other reason is that material goods are transitory. At some point in time, no matter how large an estate, it will be consumed. This was vividly illustrated in a recent documentary on the Kennedy fortune, which had been created by Joseph (Joe) Patrick Kennedy Sr., father of

John F. Kennedy, America's 35th President. The original trust fund, which was immense, has been and continues to be drained by the generations of heirs that followed Joe.

Does this mean that bequeathing wealth is pointless? Of course not. It can be a Godsend to needy beneficiaries and help assuage some of the pain in their lives. Thus, bestowing assets is a wonderful gesture.

Nonetheless, there are things other than valuables that can significantly bolster estates. The longest lasting returns can be derived from personal investments; although these appear to be insignificant on the surface, they tend to be very impactful.

And it's not uncommon to remember dead people for the manner in which they treated others while they were alive. Thus, a large component of any estate, yet one that never appears on a list of assets, is the perception of the deceased individual's character. Everyone leaves memories of who they were, a perspective by which others judge them. Perception is, of course, an inexact, subjective method to evaluate anything or anyone. Still, how humans perceive other humans becomes the reality of who individuals are when they are alive and who they were after they are dead. Accordingly, if the perception of an individual is positive, the reality of their character is positive. And the converse is likewise true. Perception becomes a permanent marker, a brand that transcends death. Long after an abusive person's death, they are likely to be poorly regarded, irrespective of the value of their estate. This brings to mind the adage, "A jackass wearing a silver saddle is still a jackass."

On the other hand, I am acquainted with prosperous individuals that are quite the opposite. One in particular, whose kindheartedness is in a league all to himself, knew how to manage his enormous wealth and his behavior. This individual is an excellent example of the value of perception. Not only has he achieved recognition because of his net worth, but he is also highly regarded for his magnanimous, underpublicized gestures. The memory of him and the life he led will be cherished long after he is dead.

And for those that desire to be well-regarded after their death, there is another motivator for them to lead decent lifestyles; modern technology makes it feasible to collect and disseminate personal information on people, removing the shroud of privacy, even after death. My wife, who is an avid lineage buff, has done considerable research on our family history using the services of Ancestry.com. She was able to gather personal records, some of which are well over a hundred years old, on a number of her ancestors and mine. As technology advances in the future, it stands to reason that obtaining such information on the lives of deceased humans will become less difficult, making it easier to research them and to shape powerful perceptions of the lives they led and who they were.

Let's get back to legacy, which is commonly considered to be the value of tangible assets. If the bottom line figure isn't the only way to measure a person's worth, what other items should be included? I can think of three: (1) contributions to mankind, (2) positive influential memories and (3) personal chronicles. All of these are prized because they potentially benefit posterity for a long time.

There is no need to devote a significant amount of time to (1) contributions to mankind. The human race rarely produces exceptional individuals like Madame Curie, Thomas Edison, Leonardo da Vinci and so forth. And for the record, Jesus Christ, who was the greatest, most influential person to ever live, was a once-in-an-eternity phenomenon that will never be replicated.

Item (2), positive influential memories, can add a great deal to the value to any legacy. I recall a famous professional golfer, who was one of the best of his era, stating that he always dedicated a portion of his time for his family. He wanted to invest part of himself to cement his relationship with them, hoping that they would know and remember him for the man he was, not for his acclaim or the tangible assets that he would leave behind. He was indeed a wise man.

I previously mentioned that my dad concentrated his life on prayer and service to his fellow man. Everybody that knew my dad thought well of him and they spoke well of him. And why not? He was always humble, never allowing his ego to drive his actions. I can unashamedly say that he is the best person I have ever known. When it came to integrity, love for his family, love for his fellow man and love for God, he set a standard that was virtually impossible to match. An honest bookkeeper for most of his career, he often rendered services to family and friends for little money, or in some cases for free. After dad passed away, I learned that he had once rendered a bookkeeping service to one of my uncles, who at the time was struggling to provide for a wife and four children. Eventually, my uncle paid my dad forty dollars in cash. Later that same day, my dad returned and gave my uncle four rolls of quarters, each worth ten dollars, with instructions to distribute one to each of the children. This story is but one small example of why I am so proud of my dad.

How would you rank the perception of the man I just described compared to that of magnate, Joseph (Joe) Patrick Kennedy, Sr., a greedy businessman whose financial accomplishments were achieved through ruthlessness and a disposition to break laws and human beings? And by the way, Joe Kennedy also committed the unthinkable act of having one of his children, who was problematic to the family image, lobotomized and institutionalized. Had you or I been an impediment in his path, imagine what he would have been capable of doing to us.

Reinforcing the value of positive influential memories is the account of Umberto Balducci, my maternal grandfather or *nonno* in Italian. He died when I was thirteen, so I didn't get many opportunities to spend time with him. Nevertheless, through stories relayed by my mom and her brothers and sisters, I came to learn all about my nonno. He was the rock upon which my mother's family was built. Here are some highlights from the life of this undereducated immigrant, who left home when he was sixteen years old with only his intelligence and workaholic ethic to overcome the challenges of survival. He sired a dozen children, who he supported with brute willpower and hard work during extremely tough times – World War I, Prohibition, the Great Depression and World War II. With the exception of Christmas Day, which he celebrated at his home, he normally worked each and every day of the year, often fifteen or more hours. Overcoming a number of obstacles, he provided for his family by being a restaurant operator, farmer and sideline real estate investor. He also sent passage money to other Italians to help them establish lawful lives in America. When he died at age seventy-two, he left an impressive estate for the time, which ended up being divided equally among his children. More importantly, his estate included lasting memories of the man he was, positive memories that bound and strengthened his family and friends. All of his children respected him, some to the point of adoration. When he was on his deathbed at home, a successful Italian immigrant that he had helped came to visit him. When the man was told his condition prevented him from knowing anyone, the man protested, "But I know *him*! I want to see *him*!" I don't know how others perceive this tribute, but that is the kind of remembrance I want. In 2017, the Virginia Department of Historic Resources recognized Umberto Balducci's villa by placing it on the only historical marker in Virginia recognizing an ethnic group.

Although I was not one of the direct heirs to my nonno's estate, he left me something much more valuable than tangible assets. What I learned about his life, in particular his work ethic and his strength in overcoming adversity, affected the way I handled myself. It was his gift to me, one that kept giving long after the material assets he bequeathed had disappeared.

As for (3) personal chronicles, this is a terrific asset to bequeath to heirs. Unlike spoken words, which can oscillate like a small branch in a breeze or can be misunderstood or misremembered, written journals are precise. There is no misquoting what was said, and such documents can endure a long time, maybe a very, very long time. And they can have a positive effect on the future. There is no better example than the writings contained in the Holy Bible, especially the New Testament. Consider the enormous impact it had on the world. As an aside, the exactness of written communiqués is the reason I prefer email or letters or text messages. There is more accountability attached to them.

Although the vast majority of humans live relatively simple existences, everyone has valuable information and experiences from their lives that could prove useful to others. Why not record them so they can be shared? The preservation of personal memoirs can take the form of something as small as notes in a diary or something as large as an autobiography; these should not be earmarked exclusively for celebrities leading extraordinary lives. In fact, an argument could be made that normal people may actually derive a greater benefit from the experiences of other normal people than they would from celebrities. Individuals lacking writing skills or access to professional writers should not be intimidated, embarrassed or easily dissuaded. The final product does not have to be grammatically perfect to be understood. And for those that have never undertaken such a project, computers and software are a big help. Even those like me that never learned proper typing technique can give it a try. If I was able to get the job done, so can others.

For those that tackle it, do it for the right reason. It should not be an ego-boosting and/or a profit-seeking undertaking. Leave that to sports stars, Hollywood personalities, heroes, politicians, tycoons and the like, people with the name recognition and the provocative, fascinating lifestyles that appeal to literary agents and publishers. Instead, personal chronicles should provide readers with facts and lessons learned that can make a positive impact on the lives of others.

Those reading this book will undoubtedly recognize that it is part of my legacy. Leaving material possessions was not enough to satisfy me. I wanted to leave an investment that would benefit posterity and pay dividends much longer than my monetary goods, something that would be educational and inspirational to others, especially to my children and grandchildren, similar to the lessons I learned from my parents and my nonno. And I wanted to do it in such a way that, when my children and grandchildren were approaching the end of their lives, they would consider leaving a legacy like mine.

In summary, the net worth of an individual's legacy, the finite part of what is left behind, can be bolstered significantly by leaving a gift of inestimable, enduring value; thus, I subscribe to the principle: *augment legacies with positive influential memories and personal chronicles.*

Chapter 11

Transitioning

Looking backwards to the time that I was contemplating entering the world of the retired, I did not recognize nor did I fully appreciate exactly what was about to happen. Simply stated, I was not properly preparing myself for the adjustment. And I'm not speaking about finances. After saving and investing for decades, my wife and I owned a comfortable, lien-free home in a beautiful rural area. We also owned IRAs, a pension account, investments and bank accounts, and we had been diligently paying into the social security fund for five decades. We would not limp into the senior phase of life without money. And both of us have conservative tastes, so we had more than enough to be stress-free financially.

I'm speaking about *time*, the irreplaceable gift that cannot be purchased at any price, the gift that is increasing, not shrinking. The senior phase of life can leave a vacuum. Before reaching it, many seniors struggle to keep up with hectic schedules that are loaded with meaningful commitments, those obligations of life that give us the essential purpose we all need. The importance of purpose cannot be overstated. It is the source of energy that propels the human engine, the motive that gives us passion for life. Without purpose, life is truly meaningless, which can induce a state of despondency, a mental condition of hopelessness.

Although I have no data to support the next statement, I believe that many seniors would be hard-pressed to proclaim a single *meaningful* purpose that keeps them going, a mission that is of utmost importance.

And I also believe that many seniors would like to devote at least part of their time to accomplish a *meaningful* objective or an agenda that gives them a sense of accomplishment and pride. I certainly wanted to continue to be productive in some way. From my perspective, stepping into this phase of life triggered a radical adjustment to my lifestyle, a result that I failed to adequately respect.

In order to make the transition as smooth as possible, I should have been preparing myself much sooner. Unfortunately, I did not. I was too close to making the move when I began to consider the magnitude of its impact on me. And the lack of planning caused me to make a poor choice, which nearly led me down a pathway to despondency.

About six months before I left the firm that acquired my company, I began to think seriously about my future after I walked out the door for the last time. I had been an industrious member of society for decades. Even if I chose to do nothing productive with the rest of my life, I had sufficient wealth to live comfortably. Certainly many people in the same position would have gladly chosen to piddle time away. Without being critical, that option was not to my liking. I wanted to do something industrious, with the caveat that it did not come at the expense of my principles or my dignity. In the end, what I chose had a hidden, hefty price tag that challenged both.

Retirement

It was previously stated that *change is inescapable*. And with regard to me, retirement was one of the most impactful changes in my life.

People can change voluntarily or change can be forced upon them. An example of an involuntary change is the process of aging, which eventually triggers the social transformation called retirement. The notion of retirement never set well with me, and I learned why after reading the definition of the word *retire*. It means to *withdraw* from office, business or active life. I consider voluntary withdrawal as an act of surrender. Not everyone accepts giving up easily. Count me as one of those.

Nonetheless, in my late fifties, I spearheaded the sale of my business to a larger firm. There were a number of compelling reasons that precipitated my decision: (1) lack of a suitable individual to take the reins of the company; (2) selling the business allowed me to recoup my investment; and (3) my business partner, who was older than me, no longer wanted to work.

After working through a five-year ownership transition agreement, which proved to be too long for me and the acquiring firm, I became excess baggage that was destined to be discarded. Not only did I not look forward to leaving my professional career, the notion was somewhat disconcerting. I didn't understand exactly why at the time, but I do now. After spending most of my life building the business, I had become emotionally attached to it. Before I sold the firm, and even after I sold it, I felt a great sense of pride whenever it achieved success. The business provided a constant stimulus for me to compete and perform, which is analogous to hitting a great shot in golf. The high goes away as soon as the ball comes to rest; there is always another shot to be hit. That challenging, endless cycle induces a powerful drive to achieve and it gives an individual purpose.

With my employment agreement rapidly expiring, I was faced with the problem of what to do. The arena that had allowed me to obtain all of those highs and had given me purpose was about to disappear. To me, retirement was a mysterious, unfamiliar concept, one that I didn't want nor did I accept. Again, I'll liken the experience to golf. Although I could no longer hit as many great shots as I once did, I still wanted to have the opportunity to compete. Unfortunately, there was no senior tour for folks in my profession.

When I was given my marching orders, I was immediately exposed to the same issues that confront others like me at the same stage of their lives. It doesn't matter whether an individual is shoved through the gate leading to the pastureland known as retirement or they walk through it. Being phased out of the work that one has been doing, even been enjoying, most of their lives happens to just about everyone: laborers, entrepreneurs, celebrities, professionals and so forth. When I faced leaving the business, I don't mind admitting that I felt lost, almost in shock. I had to grasp a harsh, but fair truth: ready or not, I was no longer considered economically viable, no longer considered fit to perform my job. Retiring was never a goal of mine. Sure, some of my acquaintances had been pointing to it long before they retired. Not me, though. I was prepared to be a cog in America's productive economy until the day I died, and I wanted it that way. Unfortunately, the world didn't see things like I did.

Without a reasonable plan for utilizing my time, this was undoubtedly one of the most disquieting, challenging situations I had ever encountered. It had been a very long time since I had tried to find something useful to do, making the experience essentially new to me. Money and time were available to me, giving me options. One of them was a lifestyle of leisurely pursuits. I knew other retired folks that seemed to enjoy working their way through bucket lists, travelling, golf, fishing and so forth.

In my case, a completely leisurely way of life was unacceptable. I wasn't interested in going anywhere that required extensive travelling. I had ventured to prominent places around the world, and I grew to abhor those trips back and forth, some of which proved to be dreadful ordeals. Even the impressive sights I had seen, like the marketplace in Hong Kong and the Colosseum in Rome, bored me after the initial wow factor was over. I had also seen live performances rendered by some of the top entertainers on the planet. Perhaps I'm an oddball, but the main value I derived from such experiences was to name-drop about my adventures in casual conversations. That was braggadocios behavior, of course, but I was just emulating everyone else. I did enjoy an occasional round of golf, but I could never spend an inordinate amount of time playing the game. Likewise, spending more than a few hours a day watching TV or reading wasn't for me. All in all, an existence totally devoid of work would not satisfy me. My high-energy persona demanded that I remain productive.

There were only a few possible options to consider: (1) volunteer my services for free to some deserving enterprise or (2) extend my career by landing a full-time or part-time position with another firm or (3) create a new business opportunity, an entrepreneurial challenge that I could conquer.

Volunteering

From my perspective, individuals that provide free services to worthy endeavors are conducting themselves nobly. Should I have chosen that option, it could have sated my need to feel useful. And it wasn't difficult to find deserving hospitals and churches in my area that sought volunteers. There were also individuals in my area that needed free help. One of my friends was providing transportation for blind people in need of access to medical providers, grocery stores and other services.

I had plenty of experience helping the elderly. While my parents were living with my wife and me, about a year before they died, my dad lost his ability to drive. My wife and I made certain they had access to everything they needed, and it was gratifying to know we were helping them. However, we did it because they were family and we felt it was our duty. Volunteering my time to help strangers was an entirely different matter. I quickly excluded it as a viable option. At that point in my life, I was too self-centered to give away *my* precious time. But life is fascinating. One never knows what is just around the corner. I had no idea, but my attitude would change.

SHOULD I GET ANOTHER JOB?
It is easier and far less risky to work for a well-established firm than to start a business. Thus, I considered looking for a full-time or a part-time job. As far as pursuing an opportunity outside of engineering, that was entirely out of the question. If I got a job, it would have to be in the engineering field, the profession I had practiced most of my career. However, it did not take long to eliminate that as an acceptable pursuit. In my mind, I was overqualified for the openings in my area, and I was skeptical about how my former competitors would treat the guy that had been locking horns with them for decades.

And there was another major obstacle in the way. Most seniors, even those with excellent credentials that are highly motivated, usually encounter bias and resistance, if not unadulterated rejection when seeking respectable employment. The acumen that older folks have harvested from experience is often overlooked in the job market. Experience should count for something, shouldn't it? There is at least one prominent person that thought so. A reporter asked this famous actress, who had just turned fifty, "Would you like to be twenty-one again?" She responded, "Only if I can bring my fifty-year old brain with me."

Like the situation with most retirees, fifty had been in my rearview mirror for quite some time. Although my brain was clicking on all cylinders, I realized that prospective employers would look at my age first, and that would be that. It is perfectly natural for younger generations to use this criterion to judge potential. Seniors are viewed negatively, seen as people that have exceeded their usefulness. Certainly, seniors have lost the blazing fastball that was once in their arsenals, but they may still have an effective slider they can consistently deliver to the corners of the plate. They just need a chance to showcase their stuff in jobs other than minimum wage positions for which most are vastly overqualified. It won't be easy to change the cultural mindset, though. Seniors must prove their merit.

And I completely understood the viewpoint of prospective employers with regard to seniors. Why should they take the gamble? The odds of making a better hire, one that will pay larger and longer returns, favors younger employees.

Nevertheless, there are a number of excellent reasons to put qualified seniors in suitable positions. We've already talked about the wisdom seniors possess. In addition, they tend to be stable, dedicated and loyal. And most of them aren't financially needy, so their talents are often available at very favorable rates.

By the way, discrimination against seniors isn't restricted to younger generations. This philosophy is also perpetuated by senior businesspersons, who believe higher profits can be achieved by squeezing work from a young labor force instead of an old one.

That said, I am familiar with one senior executive, the CEO of a successful electrical contracting company in my area that defied the odds. And he was handsomely rewarded for his gamble, proving himself to be smarter than some of his competitors. When one of his best electricians, who was proficient in all areas of the trade, reached the senior phase of life and could no longer perform effectively in the field, the CEO moved the electrician to the administrative office to manage the company's projects. The electrician, who is now seventy+ years old, has become an important factor in the company's success. And the CEO also helped the government by keeping his key man on the company's health plan, sparing Medicare from becoming this individual's primary insurer.

Let's get back to my situation. After eliminating volunteering and looking for a job, there was only one option left. I had to decide if I had the resolve to start a new business. I had done it before, so I knew what it took.

ENTREPRENEURSHIP

When individuals are considering working for themselves, they need to do some deep soul-searching. It's not meant for everyone. To turn a vision into a revenue-generating, profitable operation requires passion, courage and probably money. And, perhaps most importantly, it requires the willingness and the capability to work tirelessly without complaint.

Nevertheless, any notion that individuals must be young to create a business is ridiculous. In the case of seniors, as long as they have the required resources, they aren't severely disadvantaged when it comes to turning a good idea into a successful enterprise. And it isn't rare for people to exit the workforce with an unfulfilled dream, some business venture that had beckoned to them but was impossible to pursue while they were providing stable income for their family. In fact, satisfying such dreams can be at the very top of bucket lists. People may have to reinvent themselves, but there is nothing wrong with doing something fresh and exhilarating. Of course, the business plan must be sound and the calculated risk must be worth the potential reward.

As an example, let's hypothesize that a factory worker, who had the passion and the talent to make excellent bread and desserts at home, is forced into early retirement. This individual could consider establishing a bakery or perhaps a delicatessen, where they could offer their baked goods to the public. If they have the necessary health and financial resources, they could assess the economic feasibility of leasing an available property in their area, a potential location capable of supporting the necessary price points and volume to return acceptable profits. If everything looks reasonable, they would be ready to make that important decision to commit to the idea or pass on it.

And becoming an entrepreneur doesn't always have to be a calculated business decision. Sometimes circumstances dictate it, as was the situation with one of my dear childhood friends. When he was approaching retirement age, he faced an unusual predicament. He had been the key salesperson in a successful manufacturer's representative firm that suddenly found itself in trouble due to a serious legal problem that faced the sole owner. When the owner left the firm, my friend was sixty-seven years old, and he was confronted with a major decision. Should he retire, work for another firm or try to salvage the business? He decided to use his know-how and his connections to revive the business along with a partner, a young man with the hands-on technical skills that he lacked. Since then, the company has added more staff, all of whom had experience in the industry and were sixty+ years old. With so much valuable knowledge underpinning the new company, it has been very successful for the last eight years.

For the entirety of my life, I rarely read books unless I wanted to learn something. Thus, I wasn't well-versed in the styles that authors used, in particular, fiction writers. Nonetheless, although I wasn't an enthusiast of reading fiction, I enjoyed fiction-based movies with drama, suspense and intrigue. I would often look for holes and/or misinformation in the plots, and I would critique the actors, screenwriters and directors. When I was in my late twenties, I became stimulated by the idea of writing a book. Unfortunately, at the time, I could not satisfy my desire to write. I was too busy providing income for my family. Consequently, for the majority of my professional career, writing remained an unfulfilled quest that burned inside me.

After I sold my company, the resulting reduction in my obligations gave me more free time. It was then that my mom provided me with the inspiration to create a novel. She had received a recent photograph of an elderly woman living in Vicopisano, a commune in the Province of Pisa in the region of Tuscany, Italy. When she saw the photo, she immediately recognized the woman as her childhood playmate during the time that she lived there, eighty years earlier. I was fascinated by mom's ability to recognize someone she hadn't seen for eight decades, and she was proven to be right. Obsessed with the story, I became stimulated to create a fictionalized account of mom's life in a book titled *Gioconda's Secret*. I plowed into the novel, and I devoted countless hours to it. When the draft was finished, I asked friends, who were serious, ardent fiction readers, to evaluate it and to give me feedback. The consensus was the book was lacking in many areas. When I looked at the book honestly, I had to agree with them. I decided not to rewrite it. I simply put the manuscript away.

My interest in writing was dormant again. Then something else happened to revive it: al Qaeda's attacks on the World Trade Center and the Pentagon. One of my colleagues, the CEO of a large engineering and architectural firm headquartered in Virginia, became immediately engaged in the rebuild of the Pentagon. Sometime after the project was finished, as I was approaching leaving my career in engineering, I was invited to attend a presentation on the reconstruction effort. While I was watching the presentation, a thought struck me, "What if al-Qaeda had planned a follow-up attack on the Pentagon?" The inspiration motivated me to return to my computer at nights and weekends to work on a suspense novel entitled *Phase II*.

Although I was engaged in writing, I was anything but seasoned and I was disconnected from anyone that could help me. I was realistic about the prospect of becoming successful in writing. Very few writers, gifted or not, ever become popular. Consequently, I didn't seriously consider pursuing writing as a new career. I still needed to find something to do with my time. I didn't want to exit life playing, collecting retirement funds and counting money.

A BUSINESS OPPORTUNITY SURFACES

While I was pondering the dilemma, when I least expected it, I received an unsolicited offer. Through a close friend, who was and still is a very successful businessman, I met an individual with whom my friend had invested money in small real estate ventures. The individual, who had a magnetic, self-assured personality, proposed that I work with him in his land development and residential construction business. The offer intrigued me. During the entirety of my career, I had been providing services for construction projects, which often entailed land development. Thus, I had plenty of experience to bring to the table. And a number of my family members, beginning with my maternal grandfather, had achieved success in real estate. I thought, "Why not me?"

I quickly accepted the offer. After a period of moderate success in the residential housing market, this individual solicited me to invest in a multi-family residential project that was well underway. He claimed that he and a group of partners had divided millions of dollars in profit from a project similar to the one he was offering me. The venture appeared poised for financial success, and I made the investment. After a brief period of time had elapsed, he then offered my friend, the man that had introduced us, and me the opportunity to become full partners in another project that was similar to the one underway. And to sweeten the proposal, two partners from the original venture and the one underway would join us; this would bring experience to the table plus financial backing, which would be supported by financial statements sent to prospective lenders. Motivated by greed, my friend and I signed on, which turned out to be the worst business decision of our lives. It wasn't long before my friend and I co-signed loans.

TROUBLE

When it was far too late, we discovered the threesome was extremely dysfunctional and severely over-leveraged. To make matters worse, they were undisciplined money managers. For example, in real estate development, profit-taking should occur near the end of a venture, when most of the bills have been identified and/or paid. Regrettably, these men ignored that guideline. Without informing affected individuals, investors like my friend and I, when the first project was far from complete, they distributed a large sum of cash to themselves. That ill-advised act left them unable to weather the impact of site problems and the onset of the Great Recession, and it triggered a domino-effect collapse. Sometime after the first project was in trouble, they began to walk away from the financial mess they had created. While two of them were pursuing personal bankruptcy, the bank took control of the first project. They left my friend and me to finance the second project's ongoing overhead, which we did. Unfortunately, there was a glut of available housing in the marketplace, which caused the price points for each of the completed units to drop forty+ thousand dollars below cost. Even worse, there was no end in sight. When my friend and I were convinced the situation was hopeless, we filed legal papers to bankrupt the second project.

It was another lesson in life about being careful when dealing with people, particularly when it comes to selecting partners. Not having their financial statements audited proved to be a huge mistake. When the smoke cleared, the collective losses my friend and I suffered approached two million dollars, of which nearly three-quarters was his. In case you're wondering, he and I remained good friends after the ordeal was over. The bad experience actually drew us even closer.

My wife and I did not lose everything. Because she wasn't a signatory, her assets and our jointly-held assets were protected. And my IRA accounts were also safe. Thus, it did not turn out to be a catastrophic event from which we could never recover. Thankfully, we could still look forward to the rest of our lives. However, it was a traumatic event, to say the least.

Lesson learned

My transition into the senior phase of life would have been much, much smoother had I approached retirement differently. If I could plan it again, I would make a major adjustment to the method that I used. In addition to planning the financial aspect, which can take decades to do properly, I would dedicate much more time to planning my lifestyle – how to use my time – after retirement. I would treat the situation as seriously as if I was about to embark upon a new career that needed to provide a meaningful purpose after my major responsibilities disappeared. I would begin my preparation no later than two years in advance and develop a realistic strategy to bring the new lifestyle to fruition. After I entered retirement, I would do my utmost to make the transition successful.

Not starting soon enough contributed greatly to the hasty decision that proved so troublesome. Life, of course, does not allow us to wipe away our mistakes. We get one shot. We either get things right or we fail.

Recovering

After being humbled by the bad experience, I had to make a pivotal decision. I was dejected over losing a portion of the estate that I had planned to leave my heirs. And I believed it was too late for a man my age to recover the losses. Still, I understood that I needed to find something to do with the rest of my life. If I didn't, I would sink into a deeper state of unhappiness. And I sensed that I had much longer to live. After all, both of my parents died in their early nineties. This, coupled with the fact that people were generally living longer anyway, gave me the opinion that I could have as much as twenty-five or more years of life. If this actually did happen, I was adamant not to waste that much precious time.

Whatever I chose to do would have one restriction, though. It would exclude any financial risk-taking. My wife and I were doing fine, but we could ill-afford another substantial investment mistake. My fiscal approach would prioritize protecting our remaining assets. I then began to purge the self-imposed burden of wanting to accumulate more wealth or to bask in the glory of personal achievements. As I began to accept the past and my current station, a significant portion of the self-induced stress in my life was being removed.

I must admit, though, acceptance wasn't easy nor did it happen overnight. When it finally did, I didn't want to think old or act old, irrespective of being in the last phase of my life. I developed the right attitude, a positive one. All of my life I had been resilient, and I was determined to keep moving forward with purpose and passion. Fortunately, I found a meaningful drive that was catalyzed by an event that will be expounded upon in Chapter 12. The incident pointed me in a most positive direction. I changed for the better. I have my act together, perhaps better than I ever have. And I also have expectations, optimistic expectations. I expect to be happy and to make other people happy, and in the process I expect to reach bliss in the Afterlife.

PRINCIPLES MATTER

As I moved forward, the balanced principles previously discussed – wealth, work, morality, spirituality, fitness and legacy – all became significant factors in my life. We all have standards that drive our behavior, but most of us do not make a cognizant effort to itemize them. Although on the surface such an exercise appears to be pointless, there is a very good reason to do it. After all, our principles are really our foundation. When they are in writing, they become clearly visible, constantly reminding us who we are and who we want to be. I needed a base upon which to rebuild my life, and these qualities became the underpinning for the process. They proved to be inspirational. Without them and my resilient nature to prop me, there is no doubt that I would have been in serious trouble.

Eventually, after applying these principles, I developed four practices – Prepare for Eternal Life, Engage Life Head On, Reconcile the Past and Stay Fit – that would sustain me until I stopped breathing. Of course, adopting new practices is never easy. My blueprint was good, though, and I was determined to execute it.

Accomplishment

After embracing this mission, I realized that my ultimate success would be determined as much by my follow-through as my plan. I first heard this expressed by a well-respected entrepreneur, who was being interviewed about her secrets to success. I can't recall her name, but I'll never forget the key point she made with regard to accomplishment. To paraphrase her, "I'll take a plan that is 10% well-founded and 90% well-implemented over one that is 90% well-founded and 10% well-implemented." She was not discounting the importance of planning. Instead, she was emphasizing the value of execution.

Although she was speaking about business success, her point applies to other areas of life as well. When humans conceive what they could do or they should do, the notions in and of themselves are utterly valueless without the tenacity and the resources to implement them, most especially the tenacity.

Chapter 12

Practice: Prepare for Eternal Life

Prepare for Eternal Life. Sounds simple, doesn't it? However, when the topic is Eternal Life, nothing is simple. In a previous chapter, I admitted that I had equivocated on the reality of life after death. Perhaps the notion was simply too enormous for my brain to absorb. Or perhaps my ego would not permit me to accept anything vastly larger than me. Ultimately, after concluding that life after death was real, obtaining peace of mind became much easier.

A life-altering event made an enormous impact on my way of thinking. At that time in my life, I wasn't an active churchgoer. Nevertheless, I routinely got up early on Sundays just like any other day. I preferred to write in the early morning hours, because the stillness and the solitude were ideal for unsullied concentration, an essential element for any writer. And, of course, my brain was usually fresh after a night's rest.

On a random Sunday morning, after getting out of bed, I fed our dog Chispa (Spanish for Little Bit) and I exercised her in the backyard. After returning to the house, I made a pot of coffee and prepared a light breakfast. When I finished the meal, I went to the room where I wrote. I turned on my laptop and I began to think. It wasn't long before I was typing on the keyboard, creating a novel based on a few facts taken from the real estate ordeal.

After several hours had elapsed, I decided to take a break. I powered on the television set, not thinking about anything in particular. After flipping mindlessly through the TV guide, my eyes converged on a channel broadcasting a live mass. More out of curiosity than anything else, I decided to watch the program until I was ready to work on the plot again. It turned out to be a defining moment in my life. I quickly became captivated by what I was witnessing and ended up watching the entire mass. Not long after the service ended, I became inspired to initiate a major rewrite to the novel. When I completed the manuscript, it had a new title, *Homily of Change: Reawaking*, a new meaning and a new purpose.

If you're interested in knowing what would cause me to make such sweeping changes, it was the potency of the sermon given by the priest, an inspirational man I had never seen before or since. In my faith we believe in the Trinity, one God in three Divine Persons: God the Father, God the Son (Jesus Christ) and the Holy Spirit. That morning, the Holy Spirit seemed to be using that priest to reach my soul.

During those days, I wasn't easily impressed by spoken words, especially from ministers, so it was unexpected behavior for me to be moved so forcefully. As the priest spoke, I began to reexamine my mission in life. After the priest finished the sermon, a lecture on Salvation and Eternal Life, it was as though God had spoken directly to me. Perhaps He had guided me to take the break to watch this mass, wanting the priest to hand me an assignment via a subconscious message. Whether or not God was actually moving me, I concluded the project I had been working on so diligently was inadequate; I needed to reach for a higher goal.

For those wondering what this priest said that affected me so profoundly, the ensuing paragraphs, which are extracted from a chapter in *Homily of Change: Reawakening*, will provide insight. They represent a paraphrased, extrapolated version of the priest's message that was compiled from mental notes.

"The gift of life is truly special, my dear friends. With it we have been granted the chance to earn eternal bliss with God. He gave us that chance by sending Jesus Christ to redeem us. The mortal life of Jesus and His agonizing death on the cross are the manifestation of God's infinite love for us. We shouldn't, indeed we mustn't, reject it. God expects us to live good and decent lives. Life is a test. It takes tremendous sacrifice and discipline to overcome the corporeal temptations of a world replete with diversions. Nonetheless, that is precisely what God expects us to do to reach Eternal Life. Not one of us is perfect, yet we have been challenged to constantly strive for perfection. Do you acknowledge your weaknesses? Do you resist temptation, or do you give way to it?

"Loving God is mutually exclusive with self-adoration, placing oneself on a pedestal. He must be the most important part of our lives. He should be held above everything – family, friends, jobs, possessions. Yet most of us hold back something. It might be a little or it might be a lot. We become distracted, absorbed by the trappings of the world and our self-centered nature. We give our Maker something less than He expects. Most of us know what we've withheld from Him. Our conscience tells us. Perhaps it's something small like offending someone and refusing to apologize or not forgiving someone who has been offensive to you? After all, it takes great willpower to give up the natural urge to retaliate, to hate. Perhaps there is something bigger that is bothering you, coming between you and God . . . living a lie . . . or having committed a crime and not making restitution? If you have and you think you're getting away with it, you're not. Nobody escapes their judgment day. Perhaps you think it's acceptable to cheat on your spouse or to gouge customers in your business?

Perhaps you undermine your coworkers, your fellow man for self-gain? Perhaps you're a slacker, not fully giving your time and talent? Perhaps you're judgmental or bigoted? Perhaps you misuse the good fortune that God has given you? What does your conscience tell you? Is there anything you know about yourself that is unacceptable to God but hasn't been rectified?

"*Let me repeat that. Is there anything you know about yourself that is unacceptable to God but hasn't been rectified? What must you do to gain Eternal Life? Somewhere inside you, perhaps buried deeply, you know the answer. It's crying out to you. Will you have the courage to do what you know you must? Are you going to overcome what's holding you back from doing right, doing what your Maker expects?*

"*You aren't in control, my friends. No human is. Celebrities aren't. The powerful aren't. Noblemen, political leaders and self-anointed elitists aren't. Nobody is as important as they think they are. Everyone dies much sooner than they think. It happens at a time of God's choosing, not ours, and our lives are short. Think about that, my friends. How relevant is anyone? We're tiny specks of dust in the grand scheme of things. God created the Universe and life within it, not humans. Make no mistake. We're here to serve God. Prayer is the tool we use to communicate with Him. It's a deliberate act of faith, a spiritual admission to Him that we acknowledge who He is and who we are.*

"*We have the capacity for behaving morally or immorally. One side of our mind tempts us to make ourselves Number One, whispering, 'Do what's best for you. It's okay to sin or to take shortcuts, especially if nobody is looking.' Wrong. Our Creator is always looking. He gave us the Ten*

Commandments, His standards for our behavior. They're not inherently discretionary or arbitrary. The commitment to follow through act by act and to do right requires strength and sacrifice. God asks us to love our neighbors as we do ourselves. Do you have mastery over your will to do so? Do you aspire to live the cardinal virtues of Christian tradition: prudence, justice, temperance and fortitude? Only you and God can answer these questions. To reach Heaven, you must account for your sins, repent and beg His forgiveness. My dear friends, will you address those things about you that are unacceptable to God, or will you leave things where they stand… will you address those things about you that are unacceptable to God, or will you leave things where they stand?"

The priest's message was perfectly clear to me. Before I gave up my mortal life, I needed to prepare myself to face God. To make myself more presentable to Him, I had to examine my conscience and work on correcting flaws that He would assuredly find. And the sands of time were running out. Although it did not happen overnight, I gradually began to look at myself from outside the box.

I found a number of unacceptable faults, the first of which was my tendency towards egocentricity. I needed to become less self-centered and more giving. This would entail a significant change in my point of view. I would have to reject my human disposition to do just the opposite.

Egocentricity, of course, manifests itself in greed, a human instinct and one of the cardinal sins. Everyone I knew, including me, placed a high priority on amassing as many tangible holdings as possible. In America, even for those leaning slightly towards a selfless nature, there would always be constant pressure to go in the opposite direction. How could it be otherwise? We are continually, methodically inundated with advertisements and temptations appealing to our inborn desire to want more and more and more.

Even the nature of bucket lists, those unfulfilled urges that many of us carry into our senior phase of life, tend to be materialistic, self-gratifying endeavors. Readers doubting the accuracy of this statement should evaluate their list, assuming they have one, from an unbiased viewpoint. By the way, this isn't intended to be judgmental. Falling in line with modern society, although my bucket list was short, it was entirely driven by selfishness; I had aspired to achieve the acclaim and the rewards of a successful author.

However, after examining my life from a different perspective, one that concentrated on Eternal Life and peace of mind instead of worldly goods, I made a radical change to my list. My life would no longer be entirely about me. Those reading this book may be thinking, "This is hypocritical. If he didn't write this book hoping to be successful, why did he?"

That would be a fair question, deserving of an honest answer. I changed my intent, my purpose for writing. I write to share my experiences with others, and most especially with family and friends, in the hopes the lessons are useful in some small way or even a significant way. I'm disinterested in personal monetary gain from my writing; in fact, I am divesting myself from personal financial reward. As for acclamation from humans, I'm no longer interested in that either. God is another matter. I hope He recognizes my work as something noteworthy. In the end, my new motivation for writing was in complete accord with my new bucket list.

The first item on my new list was to be more giving to my family, friends and community without expecting anything in return. Unquestionably, this new agenda was driven by the need to please God. I wanted to be included as an acceptable addition to whatever He had waiting for decent people. If and when I had to justify my existence, at least I could affirm to Him that part of my time on Earth and part of my resources had been used in accordance with Christ's way of life. And, while I was still alive, perhaps my new lifestyle would make me feel better about myself.

Next on my list was to begin mending some of the broken relationships from my past. During my life, I had been party to several that were in ruins and/or severely damaged. Even worse, I had been perfectly comfortable with the status quo. I was at least partly responsible for the situations, and I wanted to do my best to repair them, to heal the wounds.

There was another item that needed to be addressed. I had been disposed to have a judgmental attitude towards others, a tendency to be impatient and sometimes intolerant. I knew this behavior would not bode well for me when I faced our Creator. I began to form a new perspective, one that was more in keeping with Jesus. I began to look at all humans, including myself, as imperfect specimens of God. I would try to ignore my nature to look for flaws, content that God would take care of individuals unacceptable to Him. However, I did make a minor exception that I believed God would approve: I reserved the right to denounce evil enacted by ruthless, remorseless criminals, most particularly those engaging in violence and savagery. I felt God would give me a pass for seeing wickedness for what it is and for taking a stand against it.

The last item on my list was to correct my attitude towards my religion, Catholicism. I hadn't been a consistent churchgoer in a long time. And my wife had also stopped attending church on a regular basis.

After deliberating on my arguments against religion, it became obvious that I had been looking at the issue entirely wrong. I had directed my attention to the blemishes in my religion. Certainly, there were faults. Any religious group is an assemblage of people, and humans are flawed creatures. I needed to adjust my thinking. I needed to look past the face of my religion and see what was behind it, what was actually important. The basis of my religion is a loving God, not human beings. The church's mission is to remind its members about why He is important and to help them find peace of mind and Eternal Life through Him. Church is merely an instrument to help His grace flow to us, a means to get some preventive maintenance done on our souls, a venue to pay just homage to Him. Without devoting spiritual time each week to praise Him and to refresh His words, we are more receptive to evil.

When I finally gave Catholicism another shot, it was a fair shot, and it was almost spontaneous. It happened on a random Sunday morning. Instead of my usual routine, I got dressed intent on attending mass at the closest Catholic church, Church of the Redeemer in Mechanicsville, Virginia. I had attended a number of Christmas, Easter and funeral masses there before, and I was familiar with it. In one important way, it was an appropriate, almost perfect choice. If anyone ever needed redemption, it was me. And there could be no better place to start mending one's soul than a church named after the Redeemer. I was considering asking my wife to join me, but I discovered the timing was poor. She had been taken ill, and she needed to remain in bed. Without telling her where I was going, I left the house and drove to the church.

When I entered the sanctuary, it was half-full and more people were arriving. Before taking a seat, I surveyed the assemblage, looking for familiar faces. Although I personally knew a number of the church's parishioners, I didn't see any of them. It didn't matter. I was there to spend some time with God, not the clergy or any members of the congregation. In fact, during the service, the lack of social distractions enabled me to place all of my attention on praising God and praying for humans in need of divine help.

As the service proceeded, some of the refrains seemed to be targeted at my purpose for being there: "If today you hear the voice of God, if today you hear God's own voice, harden not your heart, harden not your heart today," and "Open my heart, Lord. Help me love like you. Open my heart, Lord, help me to love."

During the 70+ years I had been on Earth, I had attended numerous religious services and I had listened to countless words, most of which fell on my deaf ears. On that particular Sunday, it was different. I was actually listening to the messages and meditating. The thick protective wall I had built around my soul was being penetrated.

After the mass ended, I left the building. The priest was standing outside next to the exit. Before going to my vehicle, I stopped and complimented him on the service and his homily. I wasn't just being polite or congenial. It was a sincere gesture, and I was ready to become a regular attendee at mass again. After committing to change my stance on religion, I realized the difficult part was still ahead of me. But I was determined then, and I still am. My soul had to catch up on its maintenance regimen, which had been overlooked for a very long time.

Not only did I intend to become a regular at mass, I wanted my wife to join me in this new habit that we could share together. After I returned home, she asked where I had been. She was surprised when I answered, "Mass." After returning to the same church the following week, only at a different service time, I encountered several parishioners that I knew. A few Sundays later, my wife was feeling much better. And after witnessing my resolve to attend mass, she decided to join me. The experience of being there with her was wonderful; it uplifted both of us spiritually.

Since then, we have been steadfast attendees, and it is having a positive effect on our marriage, even at our age. Although we had been together almost fifty years, marriages can always use a little spiritual help. Ours was no different. We are now faithful in making church part of our routine. It has become an important new practice in our lives, one that we intend to continue until our Creator calls us.

As for the priest that steers the parish, Father Jay Wagner's teachings are in perfect alignment with my views on God, Jesus Christ, Eternal Life, religion and life in general. During one of his sermons, he described church as a *"hospital for sinners, not a hotel for the self-righteous."* That's putting the concept of a meeting place to spend some quality time with God in terms we can all understand. Because our nature is to sin, our spirits require maintenance to prevent us from straying too far off the proper path. Church is the place to do that. Pomposity impedes humans from recognizing their flaws, and those afflicted with it believe spiritual healing is for everyone but them. If there's a better explanation than Father Jay's, I've not heard it. The sincerity and wisdom of his messages come shining through, week after week, homily after homily. I hope to be able to listen to him for a very long time.

CHAPTER 13
Practice: Engage life head on

As I was going through the process of change, I began to look at myself differently. My sense of self-importance was diminishing, and I was becoming unassuming for the first time in my adult life. I was a lot calmer, more tranquil than I had ever been. And my view of others was changing, too. I began to accept others as they were, without expecting them to be perfect from my point of view nor expecting them to do things my way. With regard to my personal relationships with others, I wanted people to appreciate me, but not for the same shallow reasons I embraced in my adolescent years. I wanted them to like me because I respected them and treated them well. There is no doubt that the homily motivated me in the right direction, but so did the example set by my wife.

UT PROSIM

The concept of willfully being of service to others, an expressive practice of selflessness, was introduced to me when I attended Virginia Tech; its motto is *Ut Prosim*, a Latin term meaning *That I may serve*. This ideology is central to the university's land grant mission, and I was exposed to it for four years.

That said, lessons are not always learned well. I'm not proud to state that, after graduating, I was not a consistent follower of this rich tradition handed to me. As I made my way through life, I often gravitated towards my self-serving instinct, the survivor's mentality that many humans tend to manifest. And for the majority of the adult phase of my life, it influenced my decisions and my behavior. When I was undergoing the change during the senior phase of life, I began to revert back to *Ut Prosim* and my wife helped me.

An Inspiration

During most of our married life, my wife worked a part-time job and took care of our home. I didn't know it, but she had been keeping a secret from me. She had always wanted to get a college education, which had been virtually impossible to attain before we married and while our children were growing. When our children left our nest, the time was finally right for her to pursue that unfulfilled item on her bucket list. After completing a preliminary curriculum at a local community college, she became a student at Virginia Commonwealth University. When my wife was about a year away from getting that coveted diploma, she was faced with a difficult decision. Our oldest daughter, who was married with three children, also wanted to get a college degree. In order to provide daycare services for our grandchildren, my wife gave up her dream, that college degree she craved. And without my wife's sacrifice, the undergraduate and master degrees that our daughter ended up earning would have been extremely difficult, if not impossible, to achieve.

Perhaps topping that example of love and sacrifice was what my wife did for my parents. When my mom and dad were in their mid-eighties, they were still living independently in their home. My wife and I would visit them about once a week. We began to notice they were struggling to take care of small things around the house. Eventually, my wife approached me about inviting my parents to live with us. Given that my mom and my wife weren't particularly close, I saw that offer as a magnanimous gesture. It wasn't long before we were building a new home with an attached in-law suite.

Just before we were scheduled to move into the new house, a family crisis struck. Our oldest daughter informed us that she and her husband were getting a divorce. Shortly after that, our youngest daughter, who was living and working in Kansas City with her husband and who had recently given birth to twins, was served with divorce papers. My wife took off for Kansas, and she stayed there for the next three months to help with the newborns until our youngest daughter could restore order. When the situation was under control, my wife returned to Virginia, and she resumed daycare services for our oldest grandchildren. At that time, my parents were residing in the in-law suite, and my wife joined me in helping them as needed.

Less than a year later, our youngest daughter won a court proceeding and with it the legal right to leave Kansas with the twins. She returned to Virginia, where she was able to land an excellent job and be closer to her family. In addition to our oldest grandchildren, my wife then became a daycare provider for the twins. Then our family began to grow again. Our youngest daughter remarried and bore a third child, and my wife provided daycare services for that grandchild as well.

While my wife was helping with the care of our grandchildren, my mom fell and broke one of her hips; for the next six months, my wife provided in-house physical and emotional rehabilitation therapy for mom until she became mobile again. A few years later, my father's health rapidly declined, and he was in and out of hospitals and nursing homes. About a month before he died, my mother fell again. This time she broke one of her arms, and she never recovered from the injury. During this chaotic time, my wife was with me every step of the way. On Christmas morning, 2003, my parents were in a local hospital at the same time. At our request, the staff moved dad's bed next to mom's bed. Our last memory of them together was when they held hands in her room. A few days later, mom was discharged from the hospital to a nursing home, where she unexpectedly pre-deceased dad on the evening of December 31. The following morning, dad passed away in the hospital. I believe they were destined to never be apart for long. That's the way it should be for soulmates, and it was for them.

In Chapter 7 we established the principle *balance self-serving behavior with sacrifice*, and we said this is a matter of judgment. It would be interesting to learn how others perceive my wife's behavior. Was she too selfless? More importantly, confronted with similar family dilemmas, what would others do? There is only one place to find answers to such deep questions: the human conscience. Some people would give their all to help with such crises, while others would be inclined to turn their backs and say, "I don't owe anything. I already did my job. It's time for me to do what I want."

There is no doubt about how my wife felt. In her judgment, stepping up to the plate for her family was a duty. When she made her decision, it was the *only* thing to do. She did it without complaint and without expectation. Her willingness to volunteer her services was a wonderful example of self-sacrifice, a shining illustration of *Ut Prosim* and living the message of Luke 6:31.

LEARNING APPRECIATION

During the years I was operating my business, I had been so focused on the financial affairs of the firm that I tended to overlook the pressure my wife was handling. At some point during my venture into real estate, instead of focusing all of my attention on my issues, I started to gain appreciation for what my wife was doing. No longer taking her bigheartedness for granted, I began to change my way of thinking. I was entering the embryotic stage of embracing selflessness, which had not been a predominant trait of mine. After bankrupting the real estate venture and being humbled by the experience, I lost my swagger and with it my disposition to be self-centered. Instead, I wanted to do more for my family, especially for my wife. I made a promise to myself. I would become more like her, and the change enabled me to learn the price and the rewards of family commitment.

While my wife was handling her part-time job, I assumed her role with our grandchildren and her chores around our house. Although I was unskilled, I was more than willing to do my best. It was then that I learned the enormity of the task my wife had been undertaking without complaint for years. I began to invest in my family, making small deposits on a regular basis, which came in the form of services, not money. I applied first aid to cuts and bruises, met school buses, prepared meals, helped with homework, provided transportation for extra-curricular activities and so forth. While I was doing that, I took care of cleaning and maintaining the house, washing clothes and other tasks as they were needed. It was tough sledding at first, but I eventually became somewhat proficient in this new capacity.

The aggregate of these seemingly minor investments paid great dividends later. They formed the basis of a special association with our grandchildren. One at a time, the five eldest entered high school and got driver's licenses. Often, when the umbilical cord of dependency is being cut, grandparents are among the first family relationships to be severed. Did our grandchildren abandon us? No. They managed to carve out some time from their active schedules to occasionally visit our home, and they still do. Sometimes they are looking for advice. Sometimes they are looking for another great home-cooked meal. Sometimes they are just looking for a little love. The motives that bring them back are unimportant to my wife and me. What matters most is that they know us and they trust what they know about us.

Over the years, several of them reminded us what we mean to them with priceless notes like the one we got after giving one our granddaughters a modest gift: "…For as long as I can remember you guys have always been there. No amount of thank yous or hugs will ever repay all that you guys have done for me. You have watched me as I have grown and transitioned from diapers to now a high school graduate. You have also seen my good and bad sides and yet showered me with unconditional love. Thank you for being my grandparents, my #1 fans, and *my best friends…*"

Anyone that has ever received a similar note will understand that life doesn't get any better than this, and it is in perfect alignment with the principle in Chapter 10.

A second calling beckons

While I was active in real estate, I was quietly working on my terrorism novel *Phase II*. About a year after the draft was complete, the book was made available to the public. Regrettably, it suffered the predictable outcome for a first time author without an effective promotion plan.

From the time I entered the world of real estate until I left it, my situation had changed. After bankrupting my only business enterprise, I was left with one worthy purpose in life: tending to my family commitment. I still had available time, though, and I wanted to reverse the real estate misfortune into a positive. The answer suddenly became obvious. Using several facts from the bad experience, I could create an informative, entertaining novel. I didn't have anything to lose. My wife and I were comfortable financially. If my writing wasn't good enough to make money, that would be okay with me. And if the novel was financially successful, perhaps some of the losses my estate suffered could be recovered.

As a result, I began to refocus my attention on writing, which to date had been an unexceptional calling for me. I was again ready to share some of my experiences with a larger audience than my immediate family and friends. I was also a stickler for detail. Any story would have to be well-written, well-researched and informative, and it would need strong characters and storylines.

After I committed to writing the manuscript, I dove into the project. When I completed it, I tested the waters with a number of avid readers qualified to judge my work. Most of them returned the candid feedback I requested. After assessing their criticisms, I began to incorporate several worthwhile suggestions. While I was in the middle of the task, I saw the homily that inspired me to initiate a major revision to the draft and to retitle it: *Homily of Change: Reawakening*. The story would offer readers more than pure entertainment value. It would have a moral theme.

When I was satisfied the manuscript was worthy of publication, I sent query letters along with samples to a number of literary agents; those that answered – a number of them didn't have the courtesy to do so – declined for various reasons. Having been a businessman most of my adult life, I respected the rejections from those that responded. Risk-reward assessments are business related, not personal. I was an unknown author, an old one at that. Why should they take a chance on me? They had no easy method to measure my heart or my ability.

I blew the rejections off. I wanted to continue. I felt God had blessed me with an ability to write, and He had given me the physical and mental ability to do so. Even more importantly, writing kept my brain and my soul in tiptop shape. It also allowed me to leave future generations some of my experiences and principles, which would be a testament to my life after I died. That is why I was intent to see my work published, with or without the blessing of the literary agent world.

Instead of sending additional queries, I decided to complete a sequel entitled *Homily of Change: Another test*. After the draft was finished, I had more unfinished writing to do. I wanted my legacy to include a book that had the potential to be much more enduring than fiction works. The book would help seniors navigate the choppy waters of the last phase of their lives. It would be a nonfiction work about human vulnerability and resiliency, the era in my life that I found happiness and reached for bliss. Its principles would also apply to younger generations, including my heirs, who I hoped would use it to remember me. And there was always the possibility that the public would find it attractive, perhaps more attractive than my novels. On the wings of that inspiration, *Aging My Way: Reaching for Bliss* came to life, and I leapt into the project.

My principles are challenged

While I was in the midst of the draft, a dilemma developed unexpectedly, and it would test my commitment to my ideologies. I would have to make one of those difficult choices that life often presents. I could either turn my back on a person I barely knew or follow my principles by coming to their aid. If I chose the latter, completing *Aging My Way: Reaching for Bliss*, which was then my top priority, would be slowed for an extended period of time. If I chose the former and ignored the call for help, only my wife and I would know. The situation was an iconic predicament: follow my principles or shun them. Which would I do?

The call

The situation was rather unusual. An elderly widow in our neighborhood, a lady my wife and I first met in 1999, placed a call to our house in 2015. The contact was unexpected because we had not interacted with her since we first met her. For the most part, she and her husband had kept to themselves in the neighborhood. Even after her husband passed away several years prior to the call, her distant relationship with her neighbors had not changed significantly. That situation changed quickly when she made the call, and she kept in close contact with us over the course of the next few weeks. When she volunteered a little personal information, we learned that this woman, who was six weeks shy of her 80th birthday, needed quite a bit of assistance. She had been a diabetic since she was twelve. The disease had caused her to lose sight in one eye and had impaired the vision in the other eye. Obviously, she had lost the ability to drive. After her husband passed away, she relied on her brother-in-law for access to medical facilities and other outside services. She didn't have any reasonable alternative to depending on him. She was childless. Her sister was wheelchair-bound and also a diabetic. Her stepson, who she loved dearly, was unable to help; he was a grandfather with his own medical issues, and he lived in another state.

Although she had been relying on her brother-in-law to help her access outside services, she had maintained her independence, which she prized, in most every other way. However, as we know, life is all about change. Unluckily, in addition to diabetes, she had developed another serious health issue earlier that year. Her sister's husband had all he could handle at home, motivating her to call our house in the hopes of befriending us, people she hardly knew.

At her request my wife and I began taking her to medical appointments and shopping venues; I was also bringing her mail to her door and helping her with small maintenance chores around the house. As we began to interact with her, we discovered that she had a keen mind and an even sharper tongue. Although she had a skeptical personality and preferred complete independence, she was always appreciative to have our help; she didn't believe in charity, and she attempted to compensate us. We told her we didn't need anything and we were in a position to help. When we mentioned people should help each other and we derived pleasure from being of service, she smiled and rejoined, "I'll give you a lot of pleasure."

About a month later, the other health problem, a cardiovascular issue, resurfaced in the form of intense pain. It was then that we became even more connected with her. In fact, tending to her needs became a dominant priority in our lives. We were with her when her cardiologist stated that she needed a valve replacement, and the surgery needed to be performed as soon as possible. Prior to the surgery, we maintained close contact with her at home. When she needed pre-surgery tests, we transported her, and we stayed with her. At one point, she asked us to tend to her obligations at home – looking after the property, taking in the mail, paying utility bills, etc. – while she was in the hospital. She had learned to trust us enough to give us a key to her house. She also wanted to give us cash to pay the bills, which we refused. Instead, we would bring any bills to her for approval and then pay them. When she returned home, we would give her receipts for reimbursement.

Three days prior to the surgery, a pre-operation test revealed that she also had a major arterial blockage. She needed to be placed in the hospital immediately. During the admission process, we discovered that she hadn't updated her legal papers after her husband died. She informed us that she wanted to get the paperwork amended after she returned home, and she mentioned a local attorney that she wanted to use.

That same day, a stent was successfully inserted to eliminate the blockage. A few days later, the defective valve was replaced. After spending several more days in ICU at the hospital, she was transferred to a nursing home to convalesce, where she spent the next few weeks until she was discharged. Throughout her ordeal, we kept her sister and her stepson informed regarding her status. We hoped her medical issues were behind her; unfortunately, they had only just started.

After a week or so had passed, her brother-in-law visited her to see how she was doing. During the stop-off, she appeared to be extremely confused, and he was forced to call the rescue squad. She was transported to a local hospital, where an examination revealed exceedingly high blood sugar levels. Over the next few days, while the hospital staff was trying to manage her blood sugar, she continued to manifest a confused state of mind. As her readings gradually improved, so did her mental awareness and her ability to process information.

Still, she was destined to be in the hospital for an extended period, and her legal papers had not been updated. The day before the lawyer she requested was scheduled to visit, a staff member asserted that a psychiatrist had declared her mentally incompetent and the lawyer's visit had to be cancelled. At least in Virginia, this was entirely inappropriate; although psychiatrists can certainly render opinions on mental competency, legal determinations are the domain of judges, not psychiatrists. Unfortunately, at that time she was too weak to avail intervention options. Lesson learned: having legal papers in order is critical.

Over the ensuing weeks, we continued to visit her several times a week in the hospital; we offered our moral support, bringing her cosmetic items and the like. Then she was moved to an assisted-living facility. Over the next several months, while we were continuing to visit her, she began to regress. Ultimately, she reached the stage where she was unable to do anything on her own, and then she died.

Looking back at it now, when our neighbor told us she would give us a lot of pleasure, she was absolutely correct. It lifted our spirits to know that we stepped up to the plate when she needed us. We can look in the mirror with a clear conscience, knowing that we had done our best. And should comparable situations arise in the future, we are prepared to aid someone else.

BACK TO WRITING

It has been said that everything happens for a good reason. In the case of our neighbor, the platitude was true. The opportunity to help her could not have come at a better time. Four months after she entered our lives, when I re-focused my attention entirely on my project, the experience had provided me with a perfect example of how selflessness can be enriching. I jumped back into the project, hoping to complete the draft in a few months. It actually took about six months. After I was done, I wasted several months reaching out to literary agents. When I had enough of that futile exercise, I decided to look for another way to get my book published. The process of finding a capable publisher with the necessary staff and delivery avenues to promote my work did not take long. Should *Aging My Way: Reaching for Bliss* gain popularity, my publisher will have been just as vital to the success as the quality of the book. I still have much more to do, and I plan to get the job done. That said, engaging life head on is not all about work.

PLEASANT PASTIMES

As previously stated, people need a semblance of balance between work and play in their lives. The productive part of my retirement is counterbalanced with a healthy mix of social activities. I continue to enjoy mingling with family and friends at the dinner table and on the golf course. I also follow intercollegiate athletics, especially the competitive progress of the athletic programs at my university, Virginia Tech.

I also added a new routine, a monthly daytrip to a Maryland casino with friends. For me, gambling is all about competing, not striking it rich. I set modest limits on losing and winning, and I stay the course. Initially, I competed against the casino at the ten-dollar Blackjack tables, where I was a slight underdog to win if I played perfectly. After spending many hours at the tables and essentially breaking even, I switched to Texas Hold'em poker. I was a novice at the game, but it was better to match wits with players than the house. I compete in limit games, which is appropriate for the table stakes I am willing to risk. The competitors are more apt to be amateurs like me, not pros on the prowl seeking pigeons to devour. As of now, I have held my own while I've been learning the art of reading people, situations and money management.

My wife and I also attend clubs with live bands to engage in something else we enjoy: dancing. We like a wide range of music and we're able to do a variety of steps, thanks to ballroom and Carolina shag lessons. We frequent two clubs in our area. Not only is dancing an excellent way for seniors to practice coordination and to get a little physical exercise, we have been blessed to meet a number of very nice people. This has been particularly true in the world of shag dancing and the time we spend at Visions Dance Club, where we developed wholesome relationships with regulars like Joe and our servers Karen and Tammy.

My wife and I also cook together . . . and at this moment I'm talking about food preparation! As I mentioned earlier, she had been the family chef before I assumed the responsibility for our grandchildren. Not long after I had become semi-proficient in the art of meal preparation, my wife retired from her part-time job. During our marriage, she had done plenty of work in the kitchen. I decided it was time for me to take over part of that responsibility. However, she decided to micro-manage everything I did in *her* kitchen. Indisputably, she knows much more about cooking than I will ever know. Not only is she a terrific chef, she's an outstanding baker. Her homemade breads and desserts, like deep-dish, Amaretto cheesecake, are second to none. Nevertheless, I was capable of making my share of tasty dishes like pork francese and chicken piccata without anybody's help. I wanted to stop her from hovering over my shoulder, but I was unsuccessful. I made a half-serious, half-joking proposition to her, "You and I should produce a reality cooking show. Of course, you would be the head chef, and I would be your assistant. Not only would the viewers learn a lot about cooking, they would be highly entertained."

Time for God

Other than worshiping God in church, I also have moments of silence when I interact with Him. When I retire for the night, I pray to our Creator, and I prefer not to approach Him empty-handed. I give Him the only thing a human can, thanks and praise for some of the many gifts He has bestowed on me: Jesus Christ, the power of forgiveness,

America, my health, my friends and my family. I also thank Jesus for giving sinners like me an opportunity to attain Eternal Life; and I ask Jesus to look after those in the world that are less fortunate than me, especially those that are ill, suffering, oppressed or lacking the necessities of life.

I also occasionally meditate on the miracle of nature. These calming times without worldly distractions allow me to reach profoundly into my soul, lost in God's wonders. I never plan them. They just happen. I recall a time from my childhood when I was alone flying a kite. After tiring of keeping the toy aloft, I wound the string and retrieved it. Then I laid my body on the ground in a horizontal position with my face up, spellbound by the sky, which had captivated me while I was sailing the kite. I remained there motionless for a few minutes, oblivious to anything other than the predominantly clear blue sky, which was the upward boundary of my world at the time. Earth was all I knew. I had no concept of other planets and galaxies, which even now are mind-boggling to me. I remember wishing to have the ability to take flight like a bird and soar as far as I dared, aspiring for the freedom to explore my environment and perhaps end up in Heaven. In that state of introspection, I was at total peace.

After I became an adult, other works of nature have summoned me to ponder the love and the power of God. One of them is the ocean. As a young man, while I was in the Pacific on a troop transport destined for Saigon, I spent a significant amount of time on the top deck of the ship. I gazed at the surrounding horizon, deliberating in peace on the seemingly endless spectacle before me and the marvels it contained. The experience calmed me, distracting my anxiety over the unavoidable danger that I was about to face. In the senior phase of my life, I continue to be awestruck by the deep sea, which is an unmatched, magnificent innovation of our Creator and tangible evidence of His existence. I enjoy listening to the rhythmic beat of waves breaking on the shore and looking at the vanishing point, mulling over the inconceivable vastness of the ocean and the countless marine life-forms contained therein. Whenever these situations occur, they elicit a relaxed, tranquil state of mind, the power of which is difficult to adequately express either with speech or with written words.

Chapter 14
Practice: Reconcile the past

When I entered the senior phase of life, I was toting a heavy burden, which was completely self-induced. During my life I had maintained a mental notepad. In it I had meticulously memorized a list of antagonists that I perceived to have offended me in some way. In effect, I had acted as a self-appointed judge and jury, and I had taken inventory of any wrongdoings. Although I had no interest in raising the stakes by retaliating against anybody, I was holding a degree of animosity in my heart.

And my list did not exclude me. I wasn't always proud of the manner in which I had treated others. Consequently, my notepad also contained a record of my misbehavior, actions and inactions that had been less than righteous and harmful to others. My conscience was bothering me. Not only was I subject to God punishing me for my wrongdoings, I was exacting my own measure of punishment via self-contempt. I was remorseful, of course, but that did not seem to be enough to assuage my sense of guilt.

I can unequivocally state that maintaining such a notepad is emotionally debilitating. Stockpiling these kinds of memories is tantamount to triggering a self-inflicted, agonizingly painful wound, one that is nearly impossible to carry through life. It is completely contradictory to the idea of peace of mind and happiness, a goal to which we should all aspire. Nonetheless, I had grown comfortable with the notion that I would have to lug this disorder to my grave. If the Son of God had to endure pain and suffering, everyone did. He had His cross to bear, and so did I. This was, of course, an entirely erroneous attitude that should have been instantly jettisoned. And it became increasingly difficult to tote such a heavy weight during the final phase of my life, even for a man with Italian blood coursing through his veins. It was a self-imposed affliction that could have been shed whenever I was ready. I simply needed to apply a little forgiveness, the fundamental ideology of Christianity that is espoused by our Creator and imbedded in this passage from the Our Father prayer to constantly remind us of the importance of clemency: "…and *forgive* us our trespasses as we *forgive* those who trespass against us…" During my life, I had said those words and heard them thousands of times, yet I seldom lived by them.

As I was recovering from the failed real estate venture, my thinking and rationale began to undergo a subtle change. It was so imperceptible that I didn't realize what was happening. Looking back at it now, I can clearly see what was stirring. I began to focus on what I needed to do to attain my goals: peace in life and bliss after I was dead. Intuitively, I realized that my list was a major obstacle that needed to be purged. Otherwise, as I moved into the future, I would never reach a state of emotional well-being.

My intolerance for people with whom I had problems, including myself, began to fade. I came to understand something that I had overlooked most of my life. Not only is it wrong to harbor ill feelings towards other humans – allow me to exclude purely demonic individuals from the ranks of humans – it is a potentially harmful, futile exercise. Like anything in life, it can go over the top, which can have damaging consequences and can cripple us. Negative emotions associated with human relationships – anger, bitterness, envy, animosity and the like – are all varieties of spiritual cancer; left unattended, they can eat away at an individual's soul until they kill it. Exorcizing such maladies is far from simple, though; and the longer they linger, the more difficult it becomes to expunge them. Therefore, they must be confronted as soon as possible, preferably immediately when issues arise that trigger them.

And based on my personal experience, the depth of the fracture in a human relationship is directly proportional to the strength of the bond prior to the trauma that caused the fracture…the stronger the bond, the deeper the break. Thus, relationships that are or that should be extremely close are susceptible to becoming destroyed. And it does not always take a major event to result in irreparable damage. In fact, such incidents can be fairly insignificant.

If I wanted peace of mind before I met our Creator, some fence-mending was in order. During the entirety of my life, my behavior and the behavior of people with whom I had relationships wasn't always exemplary. For my part in the offenses, I wanted to make amends if at all possible.

Trimming the list

Not everyone that I had offended or that had offended me was within reach. However, some of them were, including one that was extremely close…me. I didn't have the power to forgive myself for my wrongdoings. That was a matter for God, but at least I wanted to give Him valid reasons to consider the merit of my quest to be forgiven. I could begin by showing Him that I was trying to become a better man, one that He could love and respect.

Over the course of a number of years, in view of the fact that I was already in the senior phase of life and approaching home plate, I became more and more motivated to mend those relationships that had sustained damage. There is no question that my primary motive was self-serving. If I could repair them, it had the potential to make me happier on Earth and help me reach bliss after I died.

My mind began to shift into a more positive and more rational mode. I no longer rejected the idea of reaching out to people in the hope of improving our relationship, but it would be impossible in some cases. I had no idea how to find everyone, and some were already dead, including the individual that had recruited me to join the disastrous real estate venture. And I must admit that the idea of forgiving him wasn't easy to swallow at first. It was difficult to overlook his lack of remorse. Although it didn't happen overnight, I eventually released my bitter feelings and I accepted him for the man he was. And my hope is that, if he were alive and we could meet, he would accept me for the man I am.

Others I had not seen for a very long time, and I did not know if they were alive or dead. And even if they were alive, I had no reasonable means to find them. In those cases, I hoped my willingness to express remorse over any transgressions on my part that may have been harmful to them would be acceptable to God.

That said, there were several people within reach. Over the years, I could have easily tried to resolve issues, but I had allowed the situations to go unattended. It had been fairly easy to moderate my conscience with a variety of lame excuses: "I'm not the one at fault; they are," or "They should make the first move, not me," or "It's in my Sicilian DNA to feel this way," or similar self-serving pretexts aimed at tolerating the status quo. I had allowed my pride – a human failing that Satan exploits to swindle souls – to possess my spirit, to control my thinking, to take over my behavior. When a human mind gets askew, the condition is similar to an out-of-whack, manmade electronic apparatus. The first thing to try is the reset button, which often clears the problem by eliminating the state of confusion.

After I finally stepped outside the box and rebooted my brain, it began working logically again. I rejected the incapacitating feelings that had diminished my sense of well-being, which freed me to pose penetrating questions such as: "Why do I feel this way?" and "Am I making too much of it?" and "Why should I judge anybody, when that's God's domain?" The answers were simple. I had been wrong, and I needed to look for opportunities to make things right.

Love Thy Neighbor as Thyself

One of the relationships that had been shattered was with one of my neighbors. I had been living next to him, his wife and their daughter for years. My wife and I had grown to like and respect the family, and we had maintained a wholesome association with them. We enjoyed casual conversations, while respecting each other's privacy and property. This was in perfect alignment with the philosophy my wife and I have regarding healthy relationships with family, friends and neighbors. We prefer to be available if and when we're needed. And if we're not needed, we prefer to give people space.

Without warning, an incident occurred that created a breach between our families. The matter was trivial and the details are unimportant, but what happened as a result is noteworthy. Not only had the event upset my wife and me, it had also affronted my neighbor and his wife. Over virtually nothing, the fallout gained momentum and mushroomed out of control. Positions were staked out, and both sides kept the flame of discord burning. A cold war ensued between our families and the touchy relationship remained at an impasse for years.

As time passed and their daughter grew, her attitude towards my wife and I was a textbook example of how people should treat each other. It was evident to my wife and me that her parents were raising her extremely well. Despite the friction that existed between her parents and us, she was openly respectful and pleasant whenever we saw each other. It was impossible not to notice and highly admire the tacit, valuable lesson she was teaching us.

At some point my wife was ready to correct the problem. When she let me know it, I wasn't ready to bury my male ego. Satan was still exploiting my weakness. I had to serve my foolish pride, and it demanded that I remain inside my tightly-woven, uncomfortable cocoon of dysfunction. I accepted the stalemate for another year or two, and then I rebooted my brain. And there is no doubt that our neighbors' daughter and my wife were influential in helping me remove the influence of Satan on my soul. I accepted responsibility for my part, which allowed me to forgive everyone involved, including me. That was insufficient, though. I had to try to mend the damaged relationship.

One day without warning, fate intervened. I was presented with a perfect opportunity to break the standoff. While I was eating lunch with a friend at a local restaurant, I looked up and saw my neighbor seated at a table with another man. When my friend and I were ready to leave, we would have to pass their table. I intuitively knew what I should do. I needed to stop and speak to my neighbor, like I should have been doing all the years that I didn't. And that is exactly what I did, and that is all it took. Our families are now good neighbors again, and we enjoy a wholesome relationship. We don't discuss the trivial incident that caused our friendship to suffer unduly; to do so would be meaningless.

Now that it's over, my wife and I feel much better. And we believe our neighbors do too. As for their lovely daughter, she is now studying to become an attorney. As far as I'm concerned, she won her first case long before she ever thought about attending law school. God bless her for who she is and for setting such a great example.

Love Thy Relatives as Thyself

Before my wife and I were married, my tightest bonds were with relatives on my mother's side of the family. My maternal grandfather believed in family solidarity, and he passed on this principle to his children and grandchildren. While I was growing up, the family held regular reunions on Sunday afternoons. I was privileged to attend most of them. At those gatherings I came to know my mom's youngest brother, who is twelve years older than me. By the time I was seventeen or eighteen, I was establishing a strong bond with all of my uncles, including him. I came to admire his manliness, his pragmatic approach to life and his astounding cerebral capacity. As the years passed, he became my mentor.

Like me, he was an engineer. After I received my engineering degree, he helped me land my first job, a ten-month assignment before I reported for duty to serve my country. After I was discharged from the Army and was married, he and I worked for the same employer. More importantly, we also socialized together. As our connection cemented, our wives also became very close friends.

When I was in my early thirties, I cofounded an engineering business along with two outstanding partners. In time, it grew into a mid-sized firm and I became its CEO. During those years, my uncle was working for several of my competitors. Nonetheless, we remained in close social contact. For a variety of reasons, he was eventually employed by my company. At that time, he was also investing in sideline real estate deals with one of his brothers; because it didn't conflict with my business, it was perfectly okay with me. I knew they were doing quite well, and I was extremely pleased with their success.

Mixing close personal relationships and business can turn out poorly, and that is exactly what happened to us. After a long period of smooth sailing, my firm underwent a prolonged down cycle, which paralleled the construction market and the economy in general. Through a circumstantial misunderstanding, he believed that he was about to be terminated. The mix-up triggered a breach in our relationship, and we simply went our separate ways for the next twenty years. What a shame. Like the problem with my neighbors, the matter was trivial in nature, and it could have been avoided.

As the years passed, one of my cousins, who is a devout Christian man, confronted me about resolving the rift. Because I was younger than our uncle, my cousin believed that I had the responsibility to reach out. I repeatedly rejected my cousin's pleas. I didn't want to humble myself, and I was apprehensive that any attempt on my part to heal the fissure would be rejected. Nevertheless, I had been inquiring about my uncle's health, and I knew it was failing on several fronts. One of them was his eyesight. He had been born with a blind eye, and the vision in his good eye was being adversely affected by macular degeneration. Eventually, he lost the ability to drive. He became dependent on others for transportation to make medical appointments and other important matters that necessitated travel.

After I rebooted my brain, I was ready to address the issue that separated us. We had been close for a very long time, and I didn't want one of us to die with a black cloud hanging over our heads. Similar to the situation with my neighbor, without warning fate intervened. I was presented an unexpected opportunity at a funeral mass for a member of our family. My uncle was sitting next to my cousin – the one that was trying to get us together – waiting for the rite to begin. I made a point to walk past them. I stopped, shook both their hands and said hello to both of them. Because the act happened quickly and my uncle's vision wasn't good, he didn't realize it was me. After the service was over, my cousin told him what had happened. During the reception at the church, my cousin informed me the simple gesture had been received favorably. I responded that I would make myself available to my uncle if he needed me. One thing led to another, and shortly thereafter my uncle and I were sitting at his kitchen table discussing the misunderstanding that had fractured our relationship. We both regretted suspending twenty years of our friendship. With the chasm bridged, I began to help him as needed, behaving towards him like the nephew and friend I once was. We healed our wounds without leaving any scars.

I am now at peace with myself with regard to him, and I think he is at peace with himself with regard to me.

What happened to us is a classic example of how easily close relationships can become severely damaged. It is anything but rare for even minor incidents between family members to escalate until they are out of control. That ever-present force called emotion can send logic packing; and ensuing disagreements can poison relationships for a long, long time…or worse.

HONOUR THY FATHER AND THY MOTHER

Practitioners of Christian and Jewish faiths will immediately recognize this important commandment of God, which made His top ten. Before explaining its relevancy, I need to define several terms that will be used going forward. The expressions mother and father and parent(s) encompass loving human beings, who sacrifice their welfare for the benefit of their offspring. Hence, the terms exclude adult male sperm donors and/or female sperm recipients that are irresponsible and/or neglectful and/or abusive with their offspring. The term abusive does not imply *reasonable* disciplinary measures used to teach children acceptable social behavior and/or values they will need to survive as adults. I've been exposed to countless families, and I know of only one abusive parent, a male sperm donor. Like many jobs, childrearing should be judged by the body of work.

As for my parents, they were loving, kindhearted people that were never abusive, and they always sacrificed willingly to do their best for me. And I responded to the way they treated me by caring for them deeply. Long after I became an adult, I continued to have a terrific, mutually respectful relationship with my mother and father.

Four and one-half years after they came to live with my wife and me, my father began to have serious health problems. In between his periodic stays at a local hospital and a nursing home, my wife and I assisted with his care at home. When my mother fell and sustained a serious injury, it added another layer of strain. During this chaotic, emotional period, my wife and I were employed, and my relationship with my parents was undergoing a stressful transformation. When they were at home, they required constant attention, which was provided by professional sitters, my wife and me. I didn't always handle the pressure well. I wasn't always as tolerant and as selfless and as respectful as I needed to be. I also didn't take time to tell them what a great job they had done as parents, grandparents and great grandparents or how much I loved them, oversights that riddled me with guilt after they died.

It's easy to view loving parents as an entitlement, and it's far too late to show them the appreciation they deserve after they're dead. I believe in Eternal Life, yet I'm uncertain about the details of being a resident of Heaven. As far as I know, Scripture doesn't reveal if we can see and talk with loved ones in the Afterlife. To be certain of getting that job done properly, it needs to be accomplished when parents are still alive. Because I no longer had an opportunity to speak with them, I had to approach this from a different direction. I honour their memory with photos and stories, which are constant reminders of who they were and what they did and what they meant to me. I also faithfully visit their graves. More importantly, every night I include them in my prayers and I convey my heartfelt love to their spirits, hoping they can hear me.

Love thy spouse as thyself

In the world of showbiz – and books can be more than educational, they can be a form of entertainment – the top act is always the last one. Hence, since my wife is the most important person in my life, I saved her for last.

After returning to the United States from Vietnam on Thanksgiving Day, 1966, I was assigned to Fort Belvoir, Virginia. I had a few months left in service before being honorably discharged as a company grade officer. One of my duties was to serve as a member of a court martial board, which my future wife assisted as the court recorder. Almost immediately, I was struck by this stunning twenty-year old, Puerto Rican beauty. I didn't know it at the time, but she was a military brat. She was living on the Post with her mother, her five siblings and her father, a noncommissioned officer. After a few weeks, I got the nerve to ask for a date and she accepted. I quickly began to court her; not long afterward, I asked her to become my wife.

A traditionalist, she would only accept my proposal if her father consented. Because I was a commissioned officer and her dad's rank was below mine, it would make for an awkward moment. Nevertheless, it was the right thing to do, and I went to her house to beg for her hand. Her dad and I sat alone at the dining room table. I later learned that my future wife and her mom were eavesdropping on the conversation. I was nervous, but I always believed in getting down to business. He was pleasant, and he was receptive to the idea of me becoming his son-in-law. Almost immediately after he gave his permission, my future wife and her mom appeared. That was the beginning of a great relationship with her mom, whom I grew to cherish. In fact, I liked everyone in the family, and they liked me. A few months later, in 1967, we were married.

Thinking back to those days, we didn't know each other well enough to get married. Sure, we were attracted to each other, but it takes a lot more than that to sustain a marriage. To improve the odds of keeping a lifetime partnership intact, the parties must acquire mutual respect for each other, esteem that is earned over time. We didn't give ourselves a chance for our relationship to develop naturally. We entered the world of married life with a number of differences, some of which quickly became evident. First and foremost was sex. When we consummated our marriage, I discovered that she was a virgin and that she was anxious about the prospect of sexual intercourse. I wasn't a virgin, and I was thrilled to engage in sex.

Over the course of the next year or so, we discovered other incompatibilities. Each of us was temperamental, strong-willed and outspoken. My wife also began to realize that I was "old school" when it came to managing the household. As the self-appointed king and breadwinner of our family, I expected to make every significant decision, ignoring the fact that she should have an equal share of the responsibility and an equal voice in family decisions. I tried to establish my dominance. My wife, who never lacked for courage, resisted. She expected, and rightly so, to have a fundamental role in our marriage instead of the role I had in mind. Later, when I was finally man enough to admit that I had been wrong, I came to deeply regret my approach.

Although we weren't an ideal match made in heaven, we got through the rough patches. In the process, we discovered that married couples like television's June and Ward Cleaver, the Beaver's seemingly perfect parents, were rare at best. Nevertheless, we coped with our differences, like successful couples must do.

We had two daughters, who became the epicenter of our lives. During the period that we were raising our children, my wife and I cared for each other, but we still retained our individuality. One at a time, our children flew our nest. After they were gone, life became radically different. My wife and I had to establish a new relationship, and our foundation was weak. The glue that bound us together for so long was gone. We now had the opportunity to have one-on-one conversations, time to speak our minds, alone time to be honest with each other without fear of innocent ears listening to what was being said. It was time for us to look at ourselves truthfully and to disclose our faults. I had to admit that, where she was concerned, I hadn't always followed that sacred rule of life: treat others as you wish to be treated. And I wasn't always proud of my behavior. We had to consider difficult questions like: Do we love each other? Could we live without each other?

My wife insisted that we take family counseling. I didn't want to lose her. After resisting at first, I eventually agreed. While we were undergoing the sessions, I began to get an in-depth view of how my wife perceived me. I finally understood why she had been confrontational, why our marriage had at times been stormy. It wasn't easy to admit the truth: I had been a good provider and a good father, but I had fallen short of being the best husband I could have been.

If I wanted to continue life with her by my side, I needed to change. Readers know by now that significant changes can be difficult, and altering my nature was challenging for me. After retiring, although I was trying to be a better husband, I was by no means perfect. When I invested a significant amount of money in the real estate venture that failed, I made the decision without obtaining my wife's unqualified consent. She must have been a lot smarter than me; she was uncomfortable with the undertaking from the very beginning, and her intuition was proven to be right. When I realized the investment was on the brink of being lost, I had to face her and convey the facts.

It's perfectly natural for humans to be pleasant when everything is going smoothly. However, when adversity strikes, particularly when an individual's sense of well-being is under attack, their behavior is often profoundly different. Under those circumstances an individual's steadfastness, fortitude and faithfulness are put to a severe test. These moments of truth define character, whether or not people are loyal, unwavering allies or selfish, fair-weather friends. When the extent of the problem became known to my wife, she was less than pleased. Nevertheless, not only did she demonstrate her love for me, but she also exhibited her resiliency and her integrity. She passed the test with flying colors. She agreed to stick by me, no matter what that entailed. And she did exactly what she said.

Irrespective of our differences, my wife and I can look back at our life together and say the body of work turned out well. Our daughters each have their own families and successful careers. And they gave us eight wonderful grandchildren that we have been privileged to know and love.

I have never claimed to be an extraordinary judge of people. Therefore, I have to credit pure luck for being sufficiently thunderstruck to ask my wife to marry me. Irrespective of the reason, it turned out to be the best decision I ever made. She proved that she was and still is much more than a sex partner; she was and still is my best friend. As I'm approaching home plate, I'm comforted in knowing that I could not have selected a better partner to share my foxhole in life. Now, as we're readying ourselves for the slide to home plate, she and I are as happy as we have ever been. To the extent that love can be real, we have found it. We are at peace with each other.

We are almost in textbook harmony, too, but not quite. People don't easily shed their personalities, and my wife and I occasionally revert back to ours. When she is too outspoken, I like to remind her, "You need to get an inside voice, one that doesn't always say what's on your mind." When she retorts, "Hiding your thoughts is hypocritical, and I won't do it," I typically counter, "Being tactful isn't necessarily being two-faced." And I sometimes remind her of this cliché that the wife of one of my friends used: "Jesus, put your arm around my shoulder and your hand over my mouth." Whenever we have disagreements, we usually handle the situation differently than we once did. Instead of reacting imprudently, we think about how we're being perceived by each other. Sometimes we just take a deep breath. Sometimes we just look at each other and laugh. In the end, we can agree to disagree. We can express different perspectives and challenge each other without hurting each other. We aren't just life partners; we are soulmates that don't always have to be in perfect sync. We're not with each other just to satisfy our individual needs. After being married fifty years, I am as attracted to her virtue as I am to her physical presence. I love her outside and inside.

And with regard to her inside, my wife was born with a medical condition termed *situs inversus*, which is an act of nature that reverses the major organs in some humans. Statistically, she is one in ten thousand, but to me she is one in ten million. And I also beg to differ with science regarding her heart being on the wrong side of her body. I say it has never been anywhere other than the perfect place.

Chapter 15

Practice: Stay fit

Generally speaking, we seniors tend to consider ourselves to be in acceptable or better-than-acceptable condition if we: (1) have our weight reasonably under control, (2) don't have incapacitating medical issues and (3) are taking preventative maintenance drugs to counteract our disorders. Although these are vitally important and certainly factors, they are not the only variables in the equation for fitness. When I was approaching the senior phase of life, I met all three of these conditions, yet my overall health was not in good shape.

Unquestionably, in the early stages of my retirement, I began to notice that my physical capabilities had diminished. My muscle tone was melting away, and I was noticeably weaker; I could not maneuver items as easily as I once did. To make matters worse, I was losing my stamina. It was quite obvious that my general fitness was slowly disappearing, and I wanted to counteract the problem. Even if it was impossible to return to the state of fitness I enjoyed prior to becoming a senior, I wanted to impede the degeneration that was occurring. I needed a program to accomplish just that.

As stated in Chapter 9, fitness is a byproduct of a three-pronged approach. I always believed in playing the percentages; any program I undertook needed to address the Fitness Trio, but its goals and expectations needed to respect my age. I didn't want the physique or the brain of a young man. I simply wanted to hinder the decaying process.

Of course, no matter what I did, something would eventually cause me to die. I'm perfectly comfortable with the idea of death. I've had a great life, and I'm ready to make my exit whenever I'm called. However, before receiving that call, I am intent on preserving my quality of life for as long as possible and hopefully up to the instant God dials my number. This motivated me to exert whatever effort was necessary to inhibit further degeneration. At this point in time, the program I adopted has produced excellent results. Not only did I obstruct the deterioration, I actually regained some lost ground. I feel like my overall condition is better than it has been in a long time.

With that established, let's get into the details of my program, beginning with mental fitness.

Mental fitness

Exercising the brain: I use several secondary techniques to keep my brain active and alert, but my primary method is writing, which consists mostly of books. To achieve grammatical correctness, pace and storyline uniformity between word 1 and word 100,000 in a complex novel plot requires a great deal of concentration, recall and attention to detail. I devote at least three hours most days to the task of writing.

Alleviating anxiety and depression: After I sold my business, I began to experience periods of anxiety and depression. I was being negatively impacted emotionally after losing control, which induced an excessive amount of stress; I was also having difficulty sleeping. I consulted my primary care physician, who helped me get these disorders under control with medication. Later, when I was in better physical condition, my mental condition improved to the point that my periods of anxiety and depression lessened significantly and they were not as intense. And my problem with lack of rest also improved, all of which allowed me to minimize dependency on medication.

Getting proper rest: Legendary Pro Football Hall of Fame coach Vince Lombardy once said: "Fatigue makes cowards of us all." This great coach was perfectly correct, of course. And one of the factors with fatigue is lack of proper rest. The mind and the body require sleep to function up to their potential. I normally get 6 to 8 hours of quality sleep every night. Improving my physical condition and my mental outlook were important, but so was a change that I made with my TV practices. I had a habit of watching TV in bed, hoping the programming would induce a slumber that would last through the night, but this approach proved to be unsuccessful. Now I only use my bed for sleep and sex. When I want to lounge around the house or watch TV, I'm not in my bedroom. And I also try to avoid naps during the day; I want to be sleepy when I retire for the night.

Limiting alcohol & tobacco use: Although alcohol is potentially harmful to the brain, I have used various forms of it most of my adult life. At this point in time, I consume alcohol moderately and only in social settings. And except for an occasional good cigar at select outdoor social events, I don't use tobacco products in any form.

Limiting drug use: It is common knowledge that some drugs damage the brain. These include illegal recreational drugs, which I have never used nor have I felt compelled to use. Of course, I use legal drugs such as simvastatin to control cholesterol and finasteride to mitigate a urinary tract disorder. And if and when I have a kidney stone attack, which have plagued me twice, I use a doctor prescribed pain medication to relieve the intense discomfort. As soon as the attack is over, I stop taking the medication, irrespective of the number of capsules that remain; these are kept in reserve for potential recurring problems.

NUTRITION

In my experience, it is effectively impossible to out-exercise poor eating habits. This is particularly true for seniors because they normally have a diminished state of fitness, energy and sometimes health, all of which can impede the ability to exercise. Saying this another way, people, and especially seniors, need to maintain reasonable control over the quantities and types of food they eat if they hope to keep their bodies fit. And proper nutrition is also conducive to a healthy mind.

The diet I use is adequately covered in Chapter 9; there is no valuable purpose in repeating it. The plan worked well for me before I became a senior, and it still does. Certainly, it's only a guideline for me, not an obsession. If I have the urge or the need to occasionally break my diet, I have no misgivings in doing so. And I have the discipline to return to my regimen. This formula, augmented with a vitamin recommended by my primary care physician, is maintaining my weight well and providing sufficient fuel for my mind and body to function.

PHYSICAL FITNESS

When I retired, my physical exercise regimen was limited to an occasional round of golf and attending sporadic dance events. Both the quality and the quantity of these exercises didn't suit my needs. I wanted to feel better, and I wasn't getting the job accomplished.

I had been noticing several neighbors, both retired and semi-retired, walking regularly around our subdivision. Because that seemed to be a good idea, I mapped out a two-mile course in our subdivision, which included a long, steep incline. With the exception of the days when the weather was extremely harsh, I walked the course every day; sometimes, my wife would join me. When I first started, I walked at a slow speed. Gradually, I increased the level of my gait. My wife has shorter legs than me, and it became difficult for her to keep up; instead of walking with me, she joined one of her friends in the neighborhood.

Because I always considered exercise to be a work-intensive activity, not a social one, that was okay with me. Now a loner and free to set my own pace, I eventually reached the point that I was almost jogging. I wanted to take that next step, but I realized that my body would fail me. When I was in my forties and in great shape, I had been a jogger. After years of absorbing the rebound effect from hard-surfaced roads on my joints, I was forced to quit. Nearly three decades later, the effect of the pounding on my body would be much worse. As a result, I decided against going any faster.

I kept up the routine for several years until I discovered a better way to get physical exercise. When I was eating lunch with one of my friends, who is six years older than me and in terrific physical condition for a man his age, he casually mentioned something that sparked my interest. He was a member of a gym, and the dues were paid by his health insurance provider. When I asked for details, I learned we had the same insurer, United Healthcare, and the program was called Silver Sneakers. That's all I needed to hear. The program made a lot of sense to me from every angle, including economic. If seniors invested some of their time exercising, they would tend to be healthier. Therefore, they would likely lower the company's overall financial risk. Somebody at United Healthcare had their thinking cap on when they devised that plan.

When I returned home, I enthusiastically told my wife about the program; she became extremely interested because she was no longer walking with her friend. The prospect of working out in a gym appealed to her. My buddy's gym was located in a different county than our home, and we preferred joining a facility nearer to us. Later that day, I began to browse the Internet looking for a local gym that participated in the Silver Sneaker program. Before I knew it, I got a hit. There was a partaking gym less than four miles from our home.

In short order, my wife and I became members. During the orientation, we learned that the business operated twenty-four hours a day, seven days a week; members used coded cards to gain access. Thus, we could use the gym any day, any time, which was perfect. Even better, we could get our exercise without being subjected to weather interruptions and without being exposed to potentially harmful rays from the sun. We received instructions on how to use the equipment, and we were given information on the programs available there, such as group exercise classes and individual trainers. We noticed that, in addition to younger people, a number of seniors were using the facility.

When I stepped into the gym for the first time to use it, I had several goals in mind: (1) improve my cardiovascular system to increase my stamina, (2) strengthen my core muscles to moderate or eliminate periodic low back muscle spasms, which had cursed me for decades and (3) exercise and toughen my shoulder muscles, one of which had a surgically repaired rotator cuff. My goals excluded socializing with other members. Although I like people and I am communal natured, the gym was a workout venue for me, a place to maintain and/or improve my body and overall welfare. Therefore, my visits there would be primarily focused on work.

I began on a treadmill, which I used three times a week. Having never used one before, I started at a slow pace and I walked for thirty minutes. At the orientation we had been instructed on the use of multiple weight machines; several of them were designed to work the core and shoulder muscles. One at a time, I gradually added them to the treadmill regimen.

Over the course of the next two to three months, the frequency of my weekly visits increased to five or six, depending on circumstances. During that period, I also increased my pace on the treadmill from a walk to a slow jog. Eventually, I modified my gait to a fast walk on a slight incline.

I also changed my routine with the weight apparatuses. Progressively, I doubled the weights on the machines that worked my shoulder muscles. I also eliminated two machines for my core muscles. I replaced them with a slant board, and I started doing ten reps at a moderate incline. Initially, I experienced severe discomfort in my abdomen. I tolerated the pain, believing it would go away, which it did. Increasingly, I built up the routine to three sets of fifteen reps on a steeper incline. Using the slant board has worked wonders for me; the exercise has all but eliminated the muscle spasms in my low back.

Following the advice of another friend, I added two routines on weight apparatuses designed to strengthen my leg muscles. I knew his suggestion was correct because I had witnessed my dad slowly losing the use of his legs six months prior to his death. Initially, I did three sets of ten reps with small weights. Gradually, I increased the size of the weights and other settings to make my legs stronger. Lastly, I started to use free weights to improve the strength in my arms. Slowly, I increased the size of those weights, too.

Perhaps I could have continued to increase weights and/or reps and/or settings, but I wasn't in the gym to build my body. I simply wanted to have reasonable stamina and strength for a man my age in order to enjoy a good quality of life.

My wife also used the facility, but not as often as me and her workouts were less intense than mine. She preferred to walk forty-five minutes at a slower pace on the treadmill; she also used the slant board, but she did fewer reps and at a lower incline than me. Her regimen improved her stamina and blood pressure, and her cardiologist recommended that she keep up the good work.

Ultimately, I settled on a full routine three days a week, which takes about fifty minutes to complete, and a partial routine three days, which takes about forty minutes. Every routine includes the treadmill and the slant board. After I'm done, I exit the gym sweating and with a bounce in my step. The workout always gives me energy and confidence. And if I have any stress when I walk into the gym, it's gone when I leave.

Releasing those magical endorphins into my bloodstream never fails to do an admirable job of making me feel better. And the results have been substantial for my physique, too. I have considerably more endurance than I did when I initiated the program. My medical indicators have been great, as my latest visit to my primary care physician will attest. Without the use of medications, my blood pressure and heart rate were excellent. I can also use my low back and shoulders without fear, and my legs and arms are sturdier. Finally, I lost about ten pounds and an inch or two in my waist. I'm happy. My body seems to be in better shape than it was when I was fifty-five. I don't want to change a thing. I've accomplished what I set out to do, and I intend to maintain my routine for as long as possible.

And there have been other benefits to my membership. The gym has proven to be a spiritual motivator for me. Some of the members are physically handicapped. One of them is an inspirational young woman with a health problem that impairs her ability to walk without assistance. Her mother, who is her devoted companion, informed me that she suffered a severe head trauma in an automobile accident. After observing this young lady working to restore her motor functions, I was very impressed; she is the personification of resiliency and courage, a classic example of the meaning of tough-mindedness. Although she needs assistance to enter the gym and to reach the exercise machines, she does a superb job using the apparatuses once she mounts them. Whenever I feel too old, too tired, too weak, too achy or too whatever to endure my exercise program, I think about the obstacles she overcomes just to be there. Seeing her positive attitude on display encourages me to reject the fragile part of my psyche.

Although the gym isn't a social venue for me, it has allowed me to keep in touch with a number of people that I knew from other walks of life. I have also made many new acquaintances, seniors and young folks alike. Everyone there is committed to the same purpose.

We want to pay a small price to maintain or improve our lifestyles. And exercising at the gym also gives my wife and me something else we can do together.

All in all, I can't think of any good reason not to be a member.

Chapter 16
Marching forward

I believe that many of us enter the senior phase of life without a clear understanding of why we were born, without knowing our real purpose. During the adult phase of our lives, we had been accustomed to spending the majority of our time removing impediments between us and our mortal aspirations, which were almost always dictated by our innate need to reproduce, survive and prosper; we focused on achieving transitory needs that inspired us such as careers, financial gain, sex, love, acclaim to name a few. And when we reached the end, whether or not we believed we were successful, these passing aims that had dominated our existence often became unimportant.

That was certainly the case with me. During the majority of my life, I had been consumed by an open-ended series of temporary purposes, each of which had short-lived rewards. It took a very long time for me to realize that I needed to excavate more from life. After I unraveled the mystery of my true purpose in life, I had but one essential goal on Earth: reach bliss in Eternal Life. And I could look to Mark 8:36 for evidence that I was finally on target, "For what shall it profit a man, if he shall gain the whole world, and lose his own soul?" The message was clear: my earthly desires needed to be in line with saving my soul.

From now until my Maker calls me, I will continue to aspire to attain a gratifying life that does not conflict with my principal aim. My pursuits will incorporate a reasonable mix of productive work and playful diversions that have the potential to instill happiness without being at odds with my chief agenda. I will operate in this mode for as long as possible, hoping to land a spot with the souls of others that have already attained Eternal Life; I plan to exit this world knowing that I did everything in my power to become a member of that exclusive club. At this point in time, my trip is going reasonably smoothly. To remain on the right path, I must keep a few simple guidelines in front of me:

Prepare my soul for Eternal Life, by continuing to trust God and allowing my religion to have its rightful place;

Live life to the fullest, while leaning towards selflessness and tilting away from selfishness;

Do my part to promote wholesome relationships, by treating everyone as I wish to be treated and endeavoring not to judge the behavior of others (pure evil behavior aside, of course);

Stay fit, by embracing the Fitness Trio in order to retain my quality of life for as long as possible.

Now that my compass is set, I realize that my journey will be difficult. Distractions and temptations are expected in life, and care must be taken each step of the way to remain steadfast. I must concentrate on my course and be disciplined not to deviate. If and when I stray, I must make an effective adjustment immediately. And I can lean on the fact that my Creator is truly loving and compassionate; after all, He will pardon my transgressions if I approach Him with a contrite heart and ask for His forgiveness.

There is really nothing more to it than that. When my soul leaves my body, and that date is rapidly approaching, I don't want my surviving relatives and friends to mourn my passing. Instead, I want them to rejoice and remember me as one of God's miniscule creatures that, late in life, came to understand who he was and what his mission on Earth was. Remember me as a close acquaintance that sought happiness on Earth and reached for bliss in Eternal Life. Not only did he devise a workable strategy, he had the tenacity to execute it.

I have been extremely blessed for the entirety of my life. And when my situation changes, I will accept whatever my Creator has in store for me . . . both in life and in death. Humans have no choice to do otherwise, do we?